COMPLETE HOME REMEDIES

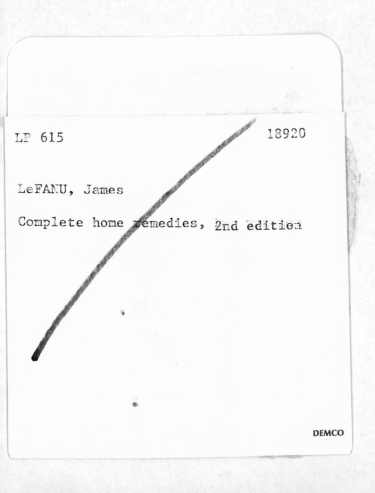

COMPLETE HOME REMEDIES

A Handbook of Treatments
for All the Family

Dr James Le Fanu

Chivers Press • **Thorndike Press**
Bath, England   **Waterville, Maine USA**

This Large Print edition is published by Chivers Press, England, and by Thorndike Press, USA.

Published in 2003 in the U.K. by arrangement with Constable and Robinson Ltd.

Published in 2003 in the U.S. by arrangement with Constable and Robinson Ltd.

U.K. Hardcover   ISBN 0–7540–8815–4   (Chivers Large Print)
U.K. Softcover   ISBN 0–7540–8816–2   (Camden Large Print)
U.S. Softcover   ISBN 0–7862–4769–X   (General Series Edition)

The text of this Large Print edition is unabridged.
Other aspects of the book may vary from the original edition.

Set in 16 pt. New Times Roman.

Printed in Great Britain on acid-free paper.

British Library Cataloguing in Publication Data available

Library of Congress Cataloging-in-Publication Data

LeFanu, James.
      Complete home remedies : a handbook of treatments for all the
      family / James LeFanu.—Large print ed.
         p.   cm.
      Originally published: 2nd ed. London : Robinson, 1999.
      ISBN 0–7862–4769–X (lg. print : sc : alk. paper)
      1. Medicine, Popular—Handbooks, manuals, etc. 2. Self-care,
      Health—Handbooks, manuals, etc. I. Title.
      RC81 .L44 2003
      616.02'4—dc21   2002028730

IMPORTANT NOTICE

This book is not intended to be a substitute for medical advice or treatment. Any person with a condition requiring medical attention should consult a medical practitioner or suitable therapist.

Contents

Preface to the Second Edition

Home Remedies was an immediate best-seller and this much expanded second edition is based on the same very simple principle. Modern medicine can do wonderful things for which we should all be grateful. Its success, however, has perhaps made us too dependent on doctors and their potent remedies. The prescription pad has sidelined the commonsensical advice of the recent past. But now this traditional wisdom has been rescued from obscurity—thanks to thousands of *Telegraph* readers. Their practical experience, past and present, of the home remedies described in these pages will I hope prove of benefit to many.

Introduction

The readers of this book will find they will save a lot of time that might otherwise be spent hanging around in the doctor's surgery or casualty department waiting to be seen. They could also save a lot of money that would otherwise be spent on medicines from their local chemist for, as will become clear, many minor ailments can be treated as easily by remedies readily available in every home. But most important of all, readers will save themselves a lot of unnecessary anxiety by learning what to do when they or their children fall victim to the hazards of everyday life— coughs and colds, sore throats, cuts, bruises, boils, skin infections and much else besides.

There is nothing cranky or difficult about the remedies in this book. Rather, they are based on a few quite elementary principles which, once grasped, make them little more than common sense.

In the past many of these simple remedies were common knowledge and so, not surprisingly, they have been suggested by those who grew up between the wars, before the great medical revolution of the post-war years. Much sound medical advice at this time was limited to advising on the use of these simple remedies which, though not necessarily curative, could at least relieve or diminish symptoms in the hope that with nature's help they would eventually get better of their own accord. Doctors no longer recommend these remedies, however, either because they do not know about them or because they believe modern pharmaceuticals are more effective.

When medicine had little to offer and many people could not afford to go to the doctor, a commonsensical approach to minor ailments was at a premium. The reason for the popularity of many of the remedies was quite simply that to a greater or lesser degree they were actually quite effective. They may indeed, as will be seen, work better or at least as well as some pharmaceuticals of the modern age and are certainly less likely to be complicated by side effects. Their wider use would also make people less dependent on medical expertise and more self-confident, and this must be a good thing.

The scientific evidence for the efficacy of these remedies is examined in the next chapter, so I will close this introduction on a personal note. I have been a qualified doctor for just over twenty years, the last ten of which have been spent in general practice. I have always been a great believer in the power and scope of modern medicine but while compiling this book I have noticed a significant change in emphasis in the way in which I practise medicine. Now, when someone comes to see me, I naturally enough reflect on whether or not one or other of the home remedies might be appropriate. I might thus advise the 'cold towel treatment' rather than prescribe antibiotics for someone with a sore throat, recommend chicken soup rather than cough medicines for bronchitis, and ice cubes rather than steroid ointments for piles.

I was initially apprehensive that patients might be hostile to the suggestion that they might try one or other of these 'old-fashioned' remedies rather than being given, as expected, a prescription to take across the road to the pharmacist. But, much to my surprise, this has not been the reaction. In a curious way I feel I have exchanged a rather mechanical style of medicine—'what's wrong, write a prescription, out the door, next one please—' for something richer, almost profounder. It is 'old-fashioned' advice, certainly, but also intelligent and commonsensical and which gives power back to the patient, so the next time round they will not have to seek my advice but rather will know how to treat themselves.

The conditions described in this book probably account for 70–80 per cent of everyday minor ailments for which the public either seeks medical advice or buys one or other overpriced proprietary preparations from the chemist. Were this notion of self-treatment to catch on widely, the potential savings on the nation's drug bill would almost certainly run into hundreds of millions of pounds.

The Evidence

There are two good reasons for being sceptical about the efficacy of self-treatment remedies. The first is the perhaps natural assumption that there is no good scientific evidence that they work—certainly when compared with modern pharmaceuticals which have been rigorously tested. Second, some remedies may seem a bit peculiar, so that it is difficult to appreciate what possible justification there could be for their use.

Neither of these grounds for scepticism is justified, as I will show in this chapter. There is much more reliable evidence than might be expected for many of the remedies, while the efficacy of the more 'peculiar' remedies turns out, on careful scrutiny, to have quite a simple explanation. This is well illustrated by contrasting the standard topical treatment for cold sores, the antiviral cream Acyclovir, with that of three alternative home remedies—alcohol, ice cubes and earwax. Acyclovir is usually prescribed by the family doctor or can now be purchased directly from the chemist for around £5. None the less, to some observers, the objective evidence for its efficacy is not impressive. Graham Worrall, Professor of Medicine, writing in the *British Medical Journal*, points out that 'Systematic review of the evidence shows that Acyclovir is not efficacious in the acute phase of an attack . . .

and that it is hardly any better when used as a preventive measure.' The doctor's prescribing bible, the *Drugs and Therapeutics Bulletin*, came to a similar verdict: Acyclovir 'confers no clinical advantage when compared to placebos'.

Now how do the home remedies compare? The herpes virus responsible for cold sores needs a high humidity to be infective and capable of multiplication—so if the water content in tissues sinks below a certain level the virus becomes inactivated. Alcohol, which in the form of aftershave, perfume, whisky, vinegar and surgical spirit is the basis of many self-discovered home remedies for cold sores, has an astringent effect on tissues, reducing their water content, thus inactivating the virus and promoting healing.

Next, ice cubes. There is abundant evidence based on personal experience that placing ice cubes for up to two hours on the site of an incipient cold sore nips it in the bud, preventing the development of the painful weeping lesion.

Finally, earwax. Earwax works in a different way altogether. Moist and dark, the ear should be an ideal place for infections of all sorts, but these are fairly infrequent because earwax contains chemicals inimical to the proliferation of bacteria, fungi and viruses, including the herpes virus. Further, earwax applied to the cold sore is the perfect material to protect it

2

against exposure to the elements and thus promote healing.

There is thus a perfectly sensible rationale for each of these home remedies and considerable anecdotal evidence to support the claims that they work. And how do they compare with Acyclovir? The simple answer is that we don't know because Acyclovir's manufacturers have never performed the necessary studies that would allow such a comparison to be made. Put another way, Acyclovir is the accepted treatment for cold sores because it was developed by a pharmaceutical company, contains a drug which is known to be inimical to viruses and comes in a tube that is sold at a chemist. Its popularity has necessarily eclipsed that of the home remedies, which have fallen into neglect because they are perceived as being 'unscientific'. This, it must be stressed, is a generalized phenomenon and applies to many of the remedies in this book. Their current neglect has nothing to do with whether modern pharmaceutical products are better; it is just that the comparison has never been made. We are dealing here with a cultural phenomenon, the ascendancy of the belief in science as the only source of reliable knowledge over traditional knowledge based on practical experience.

There is a similar sensible rationale for virtually all the remedies in this book. They turn out to fall into three broad categories, the evidence for whose efficacy will now be considered. The first category is water, whose main therapeutic properties lie in the physical effects of heat, cold and steam. The second is food and drink, particularly alcohol. Here again it is the physical and chemical properties that are important. The third category covers household items such as superglue, hairdryers, Vaseline (petroleum spirit) and surgical spirit. Finally there are the body's own secretions: one, earwax, has already been mentioned, but the secretions also include saliva and urine.

Water

Water is a chemical miracle and a biological mystery, easily the most complex of all familiar substances. Its composition seems simple enough—two hydrogen atoms flanking one of oxygen—and yet there is no simple explanation for its many peculiar properties. In the gaseous state, whether as steam or water vapour, water molecules are highly independent of each other. Yet in the solid state, as ice, water molecules interact with one another strongly enough to form an ordered structural lattice. Water is also an excellent, indeed probably the best, solvent within which all chemical compounds have a finite solubility. The many therapeutic possibilities of water depend on the effects its several different forms have on injured and inflamed tissues.

To start with, the human body is 70 per cent water, so the health of tissues is completely dependent on the conservation of water which takes place at two sites—the large bowel and the kidneys. This explains two of water's simplest therapeutic uses—in constipation and cystitis.

The main feature of constipation is a hard pellety stool that is difficult to pass, and the easiest way to overcome this is to liquefy the stool by drinking water in quantities greater than the ability of the colon to reabsorb it. 'I became very constipated when pregnant with my first child in 1956,' writes Mrs Barbara Willet from Cornwall. 'My family doctor advised "on waking every morning drink half to a pint of warm water" . . . this has worked for me all my life . . . I am seventy-five now and continue to find it infallible.'

Bacteria inflaming the tissues of the wall of the bladder cause the pain and discomfort of cystitis. The logical solution is to flush the bladder out by drinking sufficient water to overcome the ability of the kidneys to conserve it and thus increase the flow of urine.

Everything is soluble in water, and this includes the crusty nasal secretions that can be dissolved by steam inhalation—best achieved by filling a shallow pan with boiling water, placing a towel over the head and inhaling. The efficacy of this treatment has been confirmed in a study conducted by Dr David Tyrell, director of the Medical Research Council's Common Cold Unit, as reported in the *British Medical Journal.* Dr Tyrell showed that the severity of symptoms of those with a cold was halved in those who regularly used steam inhalation. Together with the direct physical effect of the steam in dissolving nasal secretions, Dr Tyrell commented that the temperature of the steam might also be therapeutically beneficial by modifying the inflammatory response of the nasal tissues to the infecting virus.

Water is an excellent medium for transmitting heat, and the next group of water-mediated therapies explores the effect of heat on tissues. When applied directly to the skin, heat dilates the blood vessels thus increasing the blood flow and with it the white blood cells that combat infection. This explains the usefulness of hot compresses when applied to styes or boils which also have the effect of bringing these conditions 'to a head' so that they will discharge their infected contents onto the surface of the skin.

When heat penetrates beneath the skin it relaxes muscles that are in spasm, and so hot baths and hotwater bottles placed directly on the site of inflamed muscles and joints are particularly popular with those who have arthritis. In addition, hot wax treatments provide wonderful relief for painful and swollen joints in the hands.

Water is also a good medium for transmitting cold, whether in the form of cold baths, ice cubes or a towel wrung out in cold water. This predictably has the reverse effect of heat. It constricts the blood vessels, thus reducing the amount of fluid that leaks out of them and so preventing the swelling of inflamed tissues. Cold also has an anaesthetic effect by blocking the action of pain fibres.

At the turn of the century cold baths—otherwise known as hydrotherapy—were a very popular treatment for a wide variety of illnesses including typhoid fever, nervous disorders and even tuberculosis. More recently, Vijay Kakkar, Professor of Surgical Sciences at London's St Mary's Hospital, has investigated the physiological effects of immersion in cold water on the human organism. He has discovered among other things that it boosts the levels of the male and female sex hormones, increases the number of white blood cells that combat infection and increases a naturally occurring blood-thinning chemical, TPA, which prevents the blood from clotting and so reduces the risk of strokes and heart attacks.

Cold—in the form of ice cubes—is particularly effective in relieving the symptoms of piles caused by the prolapse of veins around

7

the anal canal which are then pinched tight by the muscles of the anal sphincter, resulting in bleeding and intense pain. Sufferers are advised to sit naked on a chair on which has been placed ice cubes (or a packet of vegetables from the freezer) wrapped in a clean towel. The coldness of the ice cubes reduces the pain while constricting the prolapsed veins, thus reducing the bleeding from the rectum.

Ice is a similarly useful remedy for sprains and acute muscle injuries, because it reduces the degree of associated swelling. It is also helpful in the treatment of tennis elbow and similar conditions—the skin should first be oiled, after which an ice pack should be placed over the elbow for five to ten minutes twice a day.

Cold water is the definitive treatment for first-degree burns. The coldness suppresses the action of the pain fibres in the skin, while the constriction of the blood vessel prevents fluid leaking out, thus minimizing the extent of blistering.

Cold water is also a well-recognized cure for male infertility due to a low sperm count. This treatment was first described forty years ago by Dr H. A. Davidson who was inspired by a curious experiment in which scientists had placed a woolly bag over a ram's scrotum and noticed that its sperm count fell rapidly. He suggested to three subfertile men that they should do the opposite and cold-sponge their scrotum twice a day, with the result that their wives all conceived almost immediately. The rationale for this treatment is quite straightforward. A cool ambient temperature is essential for adequate sperm production, which is why the testes are conveniently placed outside the body. Thus, artificially cooling the testes further by cold-sponging or placing them in cold water should boost low sperm counts back up to normal levels.

The final therapeutic use of cold water is for the treatment of sore throats. This is indeed difficult to explain, but many people attest to it, including one of my readers whose father was a chemist. The family lived over the shop so there was an abundance of proprietary treatments readily available, but when it came to sore throats, 'a large handkerchief was wrung out in cold water, laid around the neck and covered with a woollen scarf on retiring to bed. So far as I can remember, it always worked.'

In summary, these many therapeutic uses of water give some idea of the enormous, if much neglected, potential of home remedies in the alleviation of common ailments including constipation, cystitis, boils, sprains, muscle spasm, burns, cold sores and male infertility.

Alcohol

'Alcohol is the most helpful and hygienic of beverages', observed the great French scientist Louis Pasteur. Unfortunately the general medical antipathy to this 'hygienic beverage' has meant that its medicinal properties have been neglected. Structurally alcohol appears to be very similar to water, the only difference being that one of the hydrogen atoms is replaced by a hydrocarbon. But this small difference opens up a whole vista of therapeutic possibilities, not only when alcohol is ingested but also when it is applied externally to the skin.

Alcohol's capacity to minimize and suppress the distress of cold sores has already been mentioned. In general, it is an excellent cleansing agent and antiseptic, and in the form of surgical spirit has been endorsed as a treatment for athlete's foot. Mrs Evelyn Woodford from Devon reports that 'I cured my athlete's foot twenty years ago by dabbing surgical spirit between the toes. The old skin slides off, leaving lovely healthy pink skin for ever so long as you keep off the talcum. Thereafter a daily dab of cheap eau de Cologne between the toes is all that is needed.'

Alcohol—in the form of beer—is recommended by hairdressers as a conditioner for dry hair. The suggested technique is to spray the beer on the hair after it has been shampooed and towel dried, but before it is blow dried. The smell of the beer rapidly disperses. Beer can also relieve the symptoms of constipation for the same reason as water, in that it increases the amount of fluid in the bowel, thus liquefying the stool. This effect is compounded by its sugar content, which holds on to the water thus preventing it from being reabsorbed by the colon.

The most distinctive therapeutic use of alcohol arises from its effect, when ingested, on the brain, nerves and the muscles. It provides almost instant relief from the disabling condition of essential tremor, and a small dose is an excellent antidote for muscular aches and pains around the shoulders. Alcohol inhibits the muscular spasm in the wall of the gut and has been recommended as a treatment for infant colic.

Alcohol is doubly beneficial for breastfeeding mothers (see page 65). It increases milk production, while its presence in the breast milk has a soothing effect on the baby. There is nothing to suggest that this remedy is harmful in moderation.

Food

We eat to live, but food in all its abundance and diversity has always been recognized as having quite specific therapeutic powers. It is

11

beyond the scope of this book to consider or evaluate (if it were possible) the many claims made by herbalists and practitioners of 'natural medicine' that the right sort of food can cure each and every ailment. Rather, the focus is on the specific physical and chemical properties of foodstuffs which, depending on the circumstances, can either be helpful in treating one or other common ailments, or contrariwise be the specific and often hidden cause of symptoms. Thus, as will be seen, milk can soothe an inflamed stomach but together with other dairy products may also, in some individuals, be an important cause of catarrh.

Why this might be so is best understood by considering a potato. One might think there could be nothing simpler than a potato, yet what makes a potato a potato (besides water and cellulose) is an amazing cocktail of 150 different chemicals including arsenic, nitrate, tannins, oxalic acid and alkaloids. In precisely the same way, every other type of food on the face of the earth is one vast chemical factory. Some of these chemicals, together with the physical properties of the food itself, will be beneficial by counteracting or minimizing the symptoms of an ailment in precisely the same way that the contents of a medicine bottle or a packet of pills are effective. On the other hand, some individuals may prove 'sensitive' to one or other of these chemicals and develop symptoms that can then be prevented by identifying and excluding the relevant item of food from the diet.

This 'sensitivity' takes two forms. The first is an 'allergic' reaction where the body's immune system reacts to one or other of the chemicals in the food to produce an allergic-type symptom such as the itchy rash of urticaria, the wheezy symptoms of asthma or the itchy eyes and sneezing of hay fever. These 'allergic' symptoms usually follow rapidly after exposure to the 'allergen' which allows the connection to be relatively easily made. The second form is more elusive and difficult to pin down. This is food 'intolerance', where the chemicals of one or other foods can give rise to more chronic symptoms such as arthritis, catarrh, headaches or irritable bowel. These conditions also have other causes, and it is often only by trial and error and noting that symptoms improve following removal of the culprit from the diet that the diagnosis can be made.

These two different roles of food will be considered in turn under the headings 'Food Remedies' and 'Food Sensitivity'.

Food Remedies

HONEY

Honey has been valued as a medicinal remedy from the time of the ancient Egyptians

13

primarily because of its healing properties. Indeed, there is a prescription for a wound salve from an Egyptian papyrus of 2000 BC which includes a mixture of grease, honey and fibre.

Honey is of great value in the treatment of burns and ulcers for two reasons. First, it is more effective at inhibiting the growth of bacteria and other microorganisms than many commonly used antibiotics. Second, honey is very viscous and contains the enzyme catylase which enables it to absorb water from inflamed tissues, keeping wounds clean and preventing further infection.

Dr Robert Blomfield from Chelsea observes: 'I have been using pure natural honey for the past few months in the accident and emergency department where I work and find that applied every two or three days under a dry dressing, it promotes the healing of ulcers and burns better than any other application I have ever used. It can also be readily applied to surface wounds, cuts and abrasions, and I can recommend it as a very inexpensive and valuable cleansing and healing agent.'

These sentiments are echoed by Dr A. Zimla of London's Royal Postgraduate Medical School writing in the *Journal of the Royal Society of Medicine*: 'The therapeutic potential of pure uncontaminated honey is grossly undervalued. It is widely available . . .

the time has come for conventional medicine to give it its due recognition.'

SUGAR

Sugar has similar wound-healing properties to honey. In addition, a teaspoonful dissolved in water in a baby's bottle relieves constipation. Sugar has also recently been noted to be an analgesic or pain killer, and when given to babies prior to having their heels pricked for a blood sample it 'significantly reduces' the amount of crying following the procedure.

SALT

Common salt is the most important source of sodium, which is essential for all living cells. In the thousands of years before the invention of refrigeration, salt was the main method of preserving food as it destroys bacteria thus preventing food from going off. This antibacterial effect also explains its function as a local antiseptic. Gargling with warm salt water is the best treatment for infected gums and is also useful to reduce the pain of a sore throat. Inhalation up the nose of salt dissolved in water is a standard treatment for children's stuffy noses. Adding a good handful of salt to a bidet or shallow bath and swishing around in

15

the brine provides much relief from the itchiness and discomfort of vaginal thrush.

BICARBONATE OF SODA

Bicarbonate of soda (or sodium bicarbonate) is a granular salt soluble in water and is a major component of baking powder and effervescent beverages such as soda water. It is also an alkali and so helps to relieve the burning and discomfort of gastritis caused by excess acidity in the stomach. The burning sensation of cystitis caused by acidity of the urine can be minimized, too, by alkalinizing the urine with one and a half teaspoonfuls of bicarbonate of soda in water.

YOGHURT

Yoghurt contains the harmless friendly bug *Lactobacillus* that helps suppress the proliferation of the fungal infection *Candida* in the vagina. It is advised that a pint of live yoghurt eaten each day will control the irritation of vaginal thrush, or a small amount on the tip of a tampon can be introduced directly into the vagina.

CHICKEN SOUP

Chicken soup is also known as Jewish penicillin because of the conviction of Jewish mothers that it relieves coughs, colds and other infections of the respiratory tract. In 1849, the Reverend Edmund Dixon recommended cock broth as a cure for coughs. The recipe he favoured involved running an old cock 'till he fall with weariness, then kill and pluck him, and boil him until all the flesh falls off, then strain. This broth mollifies . . . and moves the belly.'

Almost 150 years later, Dr Kumar Sakheto of New York's Mount Sinai Medical Center discovered that the beneficial ingredient of chicken soup was a sulphur compound. This increases the velocity of nasal secretions, thus minimizing the contact between viruses or bacteria and the lining of the nose. This explains chicken soup's usefulness in treating infections of the upper respiratory tract.

FRUIT AND VEG

Fruit and vegetables are an important source of indigestible cellulose that bulks out the content of the stool, thus relieving constipation. Prunes are also a potent laxative and here the vital ingredient is magnesium sulphate. Some people find that cashew nuts

17

are equally effective as a laxative, as described by Mrs Irene Evans from West Glamorgan: 'At a rather boring cocktail party, I sat near a small table on which was a saucer of cashew nuts. With nothing better to do I absent-mindedly nibbled a few. I have been constipated all my life, but next morning I had a beautiful easy motion. This was such a luxurious surprise that I tried to pin down the cause and decided it must have been the cashew nuts.'

FRUIT JUICE

The juice of the apple and the cranberry fruit have anti-infective properties. Apple juice is recommended by Yvonne Wilson from London for the infection of the eyelids known as blepharitis: 'Peel off a two-inch slice of apple, bend in half with the skin sides together until the juice appears, then place gently on the eyelids.'

There is substantial evidence that the products of cranberry juice prevent bacteria sticking to the wall of the bladder, thus making it a useful adjunct in the treatment of cystitis. Dr A. E. Sobota from Ohio comments: 'The potential use of cranberry juice in the treatment of urinary tract infections might be particularly beneficial in the management of those who suffer recurrent infections.'

Coffee and tea are astringent and reputedly an effective treatment for cold sores. Tea has other functions as well, including the treatment of blistering after minor burns. Wet teabags should be applied moist until the pain has been reduced. 'It is, of course, the tannic acid in the tea that is effective,' reports Mr G.V. Pride from Dorset. In addition, strained tea has been suggested as an antidote for eye strain.

Coffee contains the chemical methylxanthine, which dilates the airways and thus can relieve the symptoms of asthma. In a study of ten patients, Dr Schmule Kinty of the Tel Aviv Medical Centre reports that caffeine both improved their performance in tests of lung function and prevented the constriction of the airways—resulting in a wheeze and shortness of breath—that occurred with exercise.

Food Sensitivity

There are, as already mentioned, two forms of food sensitivity—an immediate reaction of food 'allergy' and the more elusive food 'intolerance' which may be a hidden cause of common conditions such as arthritis, migraine and irritable bowel. Very often the discovery is made by accident which, in the case of

Mrs O. Kabraji from Dorset, had the felicitous result of producing relief from three quite separate ailments.

About five years ago I had an acute attack of gastritis (inflammation of the stomach) which lasted almost three weeks and for which I was given the anti-ulcer drug Zantac. After reading various articles I decided to cut out all acidic fruits, red meat and dairy products. It seemed drastic at the time but surprisingly I found many enjoyable replacement foods. Anyhow, after a couple of weeks on my new diet, not only did my stomach feel better but the arthritis in my knee and back pain had disappeared! Also the catarrh that had dogged me in the winter months subsided. So in the end the gastritis proved to be a blessing in disguise.

The main offenders responsible for food sensitivity are:

MILK

Milk may cause gastrointestinal disturbances such as constipation or diarrhoea. It is implicated as being responsible for nasal and bronchial congestion with excessive production of mucus. This explains the common idea that 'milk thickens phlegm'. Other important manifestations of milk sensitivity are asthma, eczema, headache and foul breath.

EGGS

Eggs can be implicated in eczema, the itching blotchy rash of urticaria and gastrointestinal disturbances.

CITRUS FRUITS

This family includes orange, lemon, lime, grapefruit and tangerine. They too may induce eczema and urticaria and should be suspected in cases of interstitial cystitis, whose sufferers have all the symptoms of cystitis but without evidence of bacterial infection in the bladder.

LETTUCE

Lettuce is an unlikely but surprisingly frequently cited cause of food sensitivity. It has been implicated variously in back pain and sciatica, acute indigestion, irritable bowel syndrome and excess somnolence.

Further possible causes of food sensitivity include strawberries, wheat and food additives.

Household Items

Besides fulfilling their intended function, several household items to be found in every home can also double up as useful home remedies.

SUPERGLUE

Splitting of the skin at the tips of the fingers or around the heel causes painful fissures, which are colloquially known as 'hacks'. Dr J.C. Clarke from Belfast has found that these can be rendered instantly painless by the application of superglue, while Mr David Fairburn from Argyle has found that Sellotape is equally beneficial.

TAPE

Tape has been recommended for two conditions. Applied directly over the patella, it helps relieve the pain of arthritis of the knee, while strong strapping of the chest markedly reduces the discomfort associated with a broken rib.

SURGICAL SPIRIT

The two main uses of surgical spirit as a home remedy have already been noted: applied to the lips in the early tingling stage, it will stop an incipient cold sore, and applied between the toes it will cure the most intractable case of athlete's foot.

HAIRDRYER

Hairdryers have two potential uses as home remedies. First, hot air can be soothing when applied to inflamed tissues or joints, so hairdryers may be helpful in relieving the pain of arthritis or following wasp or insect stings. Hairdryers also play an important role in the treatment of severe itchiness of the anal canal and vaginal region known respectively as pruritus ani and pruritus vulvae. Dry rubbing with a towel after bathing can exacerbate itchiness in these regions, and using the hot air from a hairdryer is a much better option.

Although there is a jar of Vaseline (petroleum jelly) in almost every home, its full potential as a home remedy may not be appreciated. Vaseline when applied to the inner surface of the nostrils during and after a heavy cold prevents them from becoming sore and chapped. A Vaseline-smeared cottonbud gently rotated around the inner surface of the anus relieves the pain of piles and smoothes the passage of the stool.

Finally, Vaseline can be used as a preventive measure against cold sores 'brought out' by exposure to sun and wind. Cover the lips with Vaseline, and a trip to the beach or a day out sailing can be enjoyed without the fear that a cold sore will erupt the following day.

Autotherapy

The therapeutic value of the body's natural secretions—autotherapy—is the most readily available but also the least appreciated of home remedies. The principle is simple. Saliva, urine and earwax all contain chemicals that are inimical to bacteria and other organisms, thus protecting against infections of the mouth, urinary tract and ear respectively. The essence of autotherapy is simply to make use of this property of secretions to treat infection and promote healing.

SALIVA

Those afflicted by the misfortune of a dry mouth not only find it difficult to masticate and digest their food but also are particularly prone to recurrent infections of the mouth and gum. Clearly then, saliva must contain compounds inimical to the growth of bacteria of which several have been identified, including lysozyme that attacks the cell walls of bacteria and lactoferrin that mops up the iron that bacteria need to grow. Other compounds present in saliva prevent bacteria sticking to the side of the mouth or prompt them to come together, the better to be swept from the oral cavity by swallowing or spitting. These chemicals are all present in highest concentrations on waking, so when used as a home remedy, early morning saliva or 'fasting spittle' is particularly recommended.

Saliva can be used to treat styes and to prevent boils erupting. 'Whenever I have an incipient boil—one knows from the feel of it whether it is going to be a boil or just a spot—I apply saliva and after a couple of days it has gone,' reports Mr Bryan Evers from West Middlesex. Saliva applied to cuts and abrasions cleanses them and promotes healing —presumably explaining the origin of the term 'kiss it better'.

Mr K. S. M. Sears from Surbiton reports that saliva can help to disperse warts. 'I first discovered this remedy by nibbling away at a wart on the knuckle of one of my fingers,' he reports. After a heavy cold, the regular application of saliva on the inside of the nostrils will prevent the skin from becoming chapped and painful.

It has been suggested that animal saliva—particularly that of dogs—is even more effective than the human variety. Certainly when a dog is unable, for any reason, to lick its wounds, they tend to fester. The healing potential of canine saliva crops up in the Bible (St Luke 16: 20–1): when Lazarus was waiting at the rich man's gate to be fed with the crumbs which fell from the table, 'the dogs came and licked his sores'.

Dr Lindsey Verrier, a physician from Fiji, describes how when 'dozing at home one day after gardening with a small abraded sore on my leg, I woke to found my very small dog licking the place'. It promptly healed. Dr Verrier subsequently mentioned this to a Fijian friend, 'who told me that in villages when lads got sores on their legs from fishing, gardening and so on the old men advised them to let the dogs lick them, so as to heal them quickly'.

EARWAX

The earhole being a damp and moist place should be an ideal breeding ground for bacteria and fungi of all sorts. In fact infections of the outer ear—known as otitis externa—are quite rare because earwax, like saliva, contains chemicals that in one way or another inhibit the growth of micro-organisms.

The only therapeutic use of earwax (there may be others) mentioned in this collection is for the treatment of cold sores (see pages 86–7). It is interesting to note that the suggestion came (second hand) from a sailor; cold sores are an occupational hazard of sailors, being stimulated by exposure of the skin to the elements—particularly sun, wind and salt water.

URINE

Urine is 95 per cent water, the remaining 5 per cent being made up of mineral salts, hormones and the important chemical urea that accounts for urine's therapeutic properties. Urine is sterile and so any reluctance to use it as a home remedy is for aesthetic rather than scientific reasons.

Urine therapy is very popular in India where a conference devoted to its many different aspects takes place every year.

Former Prime Minister Mr Desai famously drank his urine every morning. Though many beneficial results are claimed from this practice, urine therapy in this book is limited to its external applications in the treatment of infection and skin conditions.

The urea present in urine is a by-product of the metabolism of protein in the body. It is an emollient that traps water in the skin, and accordingly urea is an important component of several remedies for the treatment of eczema and other skin conditions. Exposure to bricks and mortar is a particularly potent cause of occupational eczema of the hand, and bricklayers are especially aware of urine's valuable properties. 'When old houses, built with lime mortar, were demolished it was economical to pay a pensioner to "dress" the bricks for reuse by chipping away the mortar. This made the man's hands very sore, and relief was obtained by urinating on them.'

The emollient effect of fresh urine also explains why nursing mothers in the past would wipe their baby's faces with their wet nappies in the hope of improving their complexion.

It is well recognized that patients with poor kidney function are more susceptible to infections of the urinary tract, so clearly a healthy flow of urine must contain chemicals inimical to the proliferation of bacteria. The anti-infective properties of urine have been investigated by Dr J.U. Shlagel of the Tulaine University School of Medicine in New Orleans who found that urea present in similar concentrations to that found in urine was highly effective against four separate groups of bacteria. This provides a theoretical rationale for treating conjunctivitis and ear infections with a few drops of urine, as recommended by Mr Coen van der Kroon in his book *The Complete Guide to Urine Therapy.*

Finally, Dr Amanda Adler of the University of Washington describes an unusual but highly efficacious use of urine as a home remedy in the prevention of frostbite: 'While leaving school in temperatures of 35 degrees Fahrenheit below zero, a young Alaskan boy stopped to lick a handrail and was immediately frozen to it by his tongue and lip. His father attempted to free him but could not, so instead he urinated into the boy's mouth.' This did the trick, it seems, and Dr Adler commends this first-aid technique to any quick-thinking bystanders who may find themselves in a similar situation.

HAIR

There are two circumstances in which hair can be used as a home remedy. The first is to remove grit from the eye, where a small noose of hair can be used to flick out the offending

29

foreign object without fear of damaging the cornea. Hair also counteracts the exquisite pain and copious tears in those who accidentally rub the eye after touching a chilli pepper—as described by Dr Richard Roberts, a geneticist from Texas. 'I once experienced these symptoms when in the company of several Mexican friends who urged me to put hair in the affected eye immediately. Though incredulous I grabbed for my wife's hair [his own was too short for the purpose] and the pain and tears cleared immediately. I cannot explain this effect.'

Conclusion

The most striking thing to emerge from this chapter is the extraordinary scope of home remedies. Indeed, it is hard to imagine an everyday hazard or illness which is not treatable in one way or another without the need to visit the doctor or pay good money to the pharmacist.

The range of remedies is so comprehensive that it might seem difficult to remember them all, but this can be made a lot easier by thinking about them in relation to the functions of different rooms in every house. Start in the kitchen, whose ready supply of running water forms the basis of so many treatments—cold water for burns, hot water

30

for stings, ice from the fridge for piles and muscular aches and pains, boiling water from the kettle for coughs and colds. In the fridge can be found live yoghurt for the treatment of thrush, chicken soup waiting to be warmed up for bronchial conditions, and cream for the treatment of heartburn. In the food and vegetable rack are apples for blepharitis, potatoes for burns, and in the pantry cupboard, tea, coffee, salt, bicarbonate of soda, olive oil, vinegar and honey—all of which have distinct therapeutic properties. Next door in the utility room there will be a small tube of superglue and a roll of Sellotape for treating 'hacks' and a bottle of surgical spirit for athlete's foot.

Upstairs in the bathroom there is more water, this time in the form of hot and cold baths for the treatment of aching bones and joints, and a bidet full of salt for minor attacks of thrush. Here too is the hairdryer, so useful for those with an itchy bottom, and the jar of Vaseline with its multiplicity of functions. The bathroom is also the place where those so inclined might wish to test out the potential of urine therapy.

So home remedies are not quaint old wives' tales. Rather, as this chapter demonstrates, virtually all have their own logical rationale and are nothing more than the application of commonsensical solutions to simple problems.

THE SIDE EFFECTS OF HOME REMEDIES

It is perhaps natural to assume that home remedies, being simple and straightforward, do not give rise to side effects in the same way as potent drugs produced by the pharmaceutical industry. This is incorrect. No remedy can ever be guaranteed to be completely safe, though the possible hazards may be more predictable in some than others. Thus the cold compress, such as an ice cube, has many uses in the treatment of acute muscular injury, piles, cold sores and so on. There are, however, several accounts describing how overexposure can result in cold injury or frostbite to the affected tissue. So, when sensitive areas are being treated, such as in piles, the ice cube should be insulated within a couple of dishcloths and should not be applied for more than an hour at a time.

Alternatively, home remedies may give rise to allergic side effects as described in the section on nappy rash (see pages 191–2). Here the application of the egg remedy to a baby with an allergy to eggs produced an almost instantaneous widespread and violent rash. It is very difficult to give specific advice on these matters other than to urge readers to be sensible and be aware of any possible dangers.

Acne and Blackheads

Acne is the great physical misfortune of the teenage years and can, when severe, cause extensive scarring of the face. The rising levels of testosterone around puberty increase the production of oily sebum (the skin's natural lubricant) by the sebaceous glands associated with the hair follicles on the face and neck. Blackheads are small plugs of the oil which block the sebaceous gland and become black on exposure to air. Acne spots occur when the cells lining the hair follicles form a plug behind which this sebum accumulates and which then become infected by bacteria. The principle of medical treatment is first to unblock the plug; there are several preparations available from chemists, such as benzoyl peroxide, that achieve this by peeling off the top layer of skin. Second, antibiotics either taken by mouth or applied directly to the skin will attack the infection or, when taken regularly, prevent it occurring.

The following home remedies may also be useful:

Bringing spots to a head: Equal quantities of sugar and soap should be mashed together. A poultice is then placed on the spot, secured with a plaster and left overnight. The following morning once the plaster is removed the spot should have been brought to a head so it can be removed with a clean tissue or handkerchief.

Diet: It is commonly believed that several foods, in particular chocolate and fish, can exacerbate acne and so are best avoided. It is difficult to be certain of the validity of this advice, but Mrs K. R. Smith from Bedford describes the benefits of dietary manipulation for her daughter's acne: 'My daughter had very bad acne before anyone else of her age. After several years of antibiotics and creams and "you'll grow out of it" from her doctor, I took her to a homeopath. She changed her diet—no milk products or orange juice mainly—took her off the antibiotics and the result was amazing. She still had a few spots but her skin has been better ever since.'

Clean the skin: Thorough cleansing of the skin will both cut down the number of bacteria and keep the hair follicles open, as Mr H. J. Allen reports from his experience with a loofah:

> When I was a teenager my friend and workmate suffered severely with acne and his face was a mass of spots and sores. The doctor advised him to use a 'loofah' instead of a flannel to wash his face. My friend did not know what a loofah was so the doctor went to his bathroom and brought one out to show him. A loofah is

34

the fibrous part of the dried teapod of the luffa, a species of gourd. Using the loofah has a scrubbing effect and is rather painful at first but the important thing is that it stimulates the circulation and helps to remove impurities. My friend's spots cleared in a matter of weeks. I, too, used a loofah although my spots were few. Over the years I have passed on this advice to a number of young people.

Mr Eric Hayman from London suffered grievously from acne as a teenager until he realized that 'the most important thing to do was to get rid of the excess oil that caused the pores to block up and spots to develop'. This he achieved in the following way:

I reasoned that the vital thing was to remove as much oil from my skin as was sensible, and to that end I began washing myself all over with shampoos designed for people with oily hair. Such shampoos remove excess oil from the skin, especially the back, the chest and the face. As a test, after washing the back with shampoo, a thumb rubbed upwards beside the spine will not slide over the skin but moves in short jerks over the oil-free area, reminiscent of 'squeaky clean' plates. The angles between the nose and the cheeks and the nose itself should be treated to ensure the pores remain unblocked.

I realized that shampoos, etc., are not part of a doctor's normal list of treatments but they do work, the only 'side effect' is a possible over-drying of the skin if used to excess. They are readily available and are cheap and would do no harm if used in conjunction with any of the powerful drugs that are considered 'normal' in the treatment of acne.

Avoid oil-based cosmetics: This seems sensible enough, as a lot of oil on the skin will encourage acne formation.

Squeeze the spot: It is not a good idea to squeeze single pimples or whiteheads, but where there is a head of pus at the centre of the acne spot, or a blackhead, they will heal much more quickly once they are popped. To open the pores and make the blackhead easier to remove, the face should be steamed over a bowl of hot water placing a towel over the head to keep the steam in contact with the skin. Alternatively, a hot compress can be used. A cloth is soaked in hot water to which two teaspoons of bicarbonate of soda have been added. The cloth is wrung out and then applied to the affected area. Then with a clean tissue oily plugs can be gently squeezed out.

The gold wedding ring remedy, as described by Mrs Mary Goodby from Cheshire, may also be tried:

Hold the ring very firmly by its edge between finger and thumb and very slowly draw the edge of it over the chin, sides of nose and forehead with a very gentle pressure on the skin in a sort of slow motion sweeping or scraping action. Dozens of surprised blackheads and spots will pop out. The secret is to move the ring so firmly and slowly (although gently) that it hardly seems to be moving. Wash the ring and dry it well after each sweeping movement as it will be disgustingly gunged up. The pores will now look a bit odd, like lots of tiny holes, but will soon close up. Repeat every two weeks to keep teenagers' acne at bay.

Appendicitis

There is, not surprisingly, no home remedy for appendicitis. It is, however, possible to remove one's own inflamed appendix if the need arises, as illustrated by one of the few authenticated reports of a do-it-yourself appendectomy.

When the Second World War broke out, the Scottish-born Captain Robert McLaren enlisted in the Australian Army and was in Singapore at the time of its capture by the Japanese. He and a few others escaped and eventually got back to Australia. They later went back behind the Japanese lines working with the Resistance when McLaren was struck down by appendicitis. His account of the operation is as follows:

Re my appendectomy . . . I was very nauseated and had been unable to eat for a week . . . I told the locals I would have to operate. This was not received very happily, so I duly wrote out a certificate to absolve them from blame if anything happened to me.

Next the instruments were prepared in a rice pot, also swabs, etc., one castrating knife, a pair of forceps, two spoons bent as retractors, two ordinary needles, and fibre from which Manila rope is made. The operating table was two floorboards. I asked one of the locals to hold a mirror, made my incision through the skin and subcutaneous tissues, then I took the end of a spoon and spread the muscle layers, then went through the peritoneum and bared the appendix [which was] tied off and amputated. I buried the stump, spread the muscle back and sutured up. Time: four and a half hours. Healed in three days. Japs pushed in on me on day five; I took to the hills. Perfect wound.

Arthritis

Arthritis comes in many guises, though it is usual to distinguish between the 'inflammatory' type such as rheumatoid arthritis whose cause is not known and which can affect any joint, and the 'wear and tear' arthritis of ageing, osteoarthritis, which tends to affect the spine and the main weight-bearing joints of the hips and knees. Though the joints are primarily affected, the muscles and tendons may also be involved.

The range of remedies for arthritis is certainly diverse, with orthodox doctors placing their trust in drugs and surgery while complementary practitioners tend to advocate more physical forms of therapy and dietary manipulation. The difference in approach goes back to the 1950s when steroids and other anti-inflammatory drugs were found to have a dramatic effect in alleviating the symptoms of arthritis. Many doctors at the time thought these were the 'answer' and became heavily committed to drugs as the only respectable mode of treatment, dismissing any other therapy. The surge in popularity of complementary medicine, which began in the 1970s, led to the rediscovery of the traditional and neglected approaches to treatment. And nowhere was this more obvious than over the vexed issue of diet. Doctors have tended to dismiss any suggestion that food might be important, but many patients have discovered that dietary changes such as cutting down on dairy foods or increasing the amount of fish can on occasion be dramatically beneficial in easing their symptoms.

The relative merits of these two approaches are examined in a classic book, *Arthritis: What Really Works* by Dava Sobel and Arthur Klein. The authors interviewed over a thousand people with arthritis to obtain their dispassionate views, from which it emerged that in general modern medical treatments for arthritis are pretty effective in minimizing the acute symptoms of pain and swelling, preventing the progressive damage to joints and, most dramatically of all, replacing damaged joints altogether. None, however, is completely effective, and patients will always have a degree of pain and discomfort from their symptoms for which there are probably more home remedies than for any other condition. These range from copper bracelets or bee venom to thrashing the affected joints with nettles. Some of the following will be well known to those with arthritis, but those that are not may be worth a try.

Heat: Hot or warm baths twice a day are life saving for many of those with arthritis. A jacuzzi is even better for those who can afford it, and if they cannot there is always the option of paying a visit to the local health club.

Ice: Sprains and other acute injuries of the muscle are best treated with an ice pack (or packet of frozen peas) wrapped in a towel and applied directly. Heat is an inappropriate remedy here as it encourages the release of fluid from the damaged muscles which then increases the size of the swollen area dramatically. Ice packs are also an appropriate remedy for tennis elbow and similar conditions, as described by Judy Swain, a physiotherapist from Essex: 'Oil the skin and place an ice pack over the elbow for five to ten minutes, twice a day. Rest the arm but ensure you can fully straighten the elbow twice a day. If still very painful after seventy-two hours, seek further medical help.'

Towels: This remedy is very similar to that recommended for sore throats (see pages 233–4) and here is described by Pauline Casley from West Sussex: 'First wring out a towel in cold water which should be wrapped around the affected joint and covered with a woollen scarf or garment, not too tightly. This should be fastened securely in place. Then put on your pyjamas and go to bed. A gentle heat will begin to permeate the joint comforting and relieving the pain and swelling. Remove in the morning.'

Tape: The tape remedy as described by Professor Paul Dieppe from Bristol may be a useful supplementary treatment, together with 'quads' exercises (to increase the strength of the quadriceps muscle), for those with osteoarthritis of the knee: 'The principle is that the malalignment of the patella in the knee joint may cause an abnormal distribution of pressures in the knee which is corrected by placing a tape directly over the patella so that it is shifted towards the midline.' Specialist advice from a physiotherapist is probably necessary to learn the precise technique, but afterwards it can be applied regularly at home.

Massage: An instinctive reaction to any ache or pain is to massage it thus improving the circulation and bringing warmth to the affected part. Massage, preferably with the aid of essential oils, is an excellent treatment, though interestingly the results always seem much better when someone else is doing it.

Wax: Wax treatments provide wonderful relief for painful and swollen joints in the hands. This do-it-yourself recipe was provided by one of the contributors to *Arthritis: What Really Works* by Dava Sobel and Arthur Klein.

Melt a couple of packages of canning

paraffin in a tall pot to fill it about half way and then mineral oil should be added until it is three-quarters full and the mixture should be stirred well. Next the pot should be removed from the heat and left to cool until a light skin forms over the paraffin. Then keeping the fingers slightly apart dip one hand and wrist in quickly and out again. The paraffin should be allowed to dry slightly between dips which should be repeated about ten times. The hands should then be covered with a plastic bag and wrapped with a warm towel left on for twenty minutes during which time the hand should be kept still or alternatively hand exercises can be performed in the soothing heat. The paraffin should then be peeled off and saved for use another time. The process should then be repeated on the other hand and when finished the hands and fingers should be massaged with the mineral oil that remains on the skin.

Diet: Rheumatoid arthritis, like several other conditions, may be relieved or exacerbated by certain foods, though which foods are relevant for which individuals can really only be found by trial and error. Fish, particularly oily fish, is thought to be particularly beneficial, while the exclusion of dairy foods, tomatoes and white potatoes from the diet can sometimes bring dramatic relief, as illustrated by the following accounts.

Orange Juice
Mrs Angela Bromley-Martin from Sussex, 'a very active person exercising two spaniels every day and swimming twice a week', describes her experience with 'orange juice and arthritis of the hand':

> After drinking freshly squeezed orange juice with my breakfast every morning for years I gave it up. I forgot all about the arthritis. We went to stay in a hotel for a week and I had orange juice for breakfast every morning and the arthritis came back. Still it had not occurred to me there was any link between the two. Home again and the arthritis went. Three months later in another hotel, orange juice for breakfast and my hand was painful again. Then the penny dropped and I realized that the arthritis appeared to be linked to drinking fresh orange juice on a regular basis.

Mr Bernard Gudgeon of Surrey, head gardener on a private estate, read the above account with the following consequences:

> About a year or so back, I developed a sort of arthritic right hand which I put

down to my age and years of using secateurs. I also gradually developed a badly congested nose to boot, which I put down to something else, i.e., living in a dusty cottage. However, both these symptoms only occurred in the summer months, and got better in the winter which was odd as aches and pains usually get better in the warmer days. I only drink orange juice after meals and when I am thirsty. Not much in winter but about a gallon a week in summer. Then I read the article [describing Mrs Bromley-Martin's experience] and the penny dropped! I stopped taking the orange juice and within days my right hand got better and my nose cleared up! I am astounded!

Potatoes
The following account of the effect of excluding potatoes from the diet is taken from *Arthritis Today*, 29 April 1993.

The things to be avoided are all members of the family Solanaceae—green peppers, red peppers, chillies, aubergines, pimento, paprika and potato. It is the potatoes that I really do miss. As a non-cooking widower (nigh on eighty) a jacket potato is a boon. All I can say is that if I stick to the diet I am pain free and if I abandon it then within one day or at most three (if I continue to transgress) the pain in my hips returns. I don't mean maybe. Before . . . I had really to sum up determination before taking the dog for a walk my hips were so painful. Quite apart from the one and a half hours of dog walking, I play golf from time to time, and am a bit weary after fourteen holes but not in pain. It might take three to six months for the benefit to appear. In my case it was about six weeks and oh boy! is it worth it!

Cod Liver Oil

Mrs Patricia Lyon from Bristol suffered such severe rheumatoid arthritis of the hands that she 'could not turn off a tap, pour the tea or even shake anyone's hand, the pain was so excruciating'. She was under the care of a specialist, but like many people with arthritis in sheer desperation she 'looked elsewhere for help until I finally tried cod liver oil in milk'. She describes the results as follows: 'Gradually after two months the pain disappeared and also the swelling in the joints. For six months it was suggested that instead of a daily dose, once a week would maintain the status quo. This did not work for me, the pain returning and the gradual swelling of the wrist too, so I resumed the daily dose and within a week the pain and swelling went.'

Mrs Lyon describes her 'recipe' as follows:

46

'On getting up, ten minutes after a warm drink, shake together four tablespoons of milk and one tablespoon of cod liver oil to a slow count of ten and drink it up. If the lips are wiped immediately there is no taste of anything other than the milk. Then no food for thirty minutes when I have breakfast which is just a round of toast. I now have no pain, no swelling and can shake hands, turn on a tap and even wring out a cloth.'

Athlete's Foot

Athlete's foot is caused by a fungus, Tinea pedis, picked up from the swimming pool or communal washroom floor, that gets a hold between the toes where the combination of high humidity and warm temperature encourages the propagation of its spores. In no time the skin is cracked and macerated which is both painful and very itchy.

The most striking feature of athlete's foot is its intractability. Once acquired it will rumble on for years with intermittent acute exacerbation and proves remarkably resilient to the host of antifungal creams prescribed by doctors or purchased over the counter from chemists, though the antifungal drug terbinafine taken orally for a couple of weeks is very effective.

The main reason why athlete's foot fails to

respond to these antifungal remedies is that after a while the condition is sustained by various types of bacteria that take advantage of the unhealthy tissue between the toes. These in turn are responsible for emitting a variety of foul-smelling odours with names like putrescin and cadavarine.

Athlete's foot is thus an ecological wonderland inhabited by both fungi and bacteria which can be difficult to eradicate by conventional treatment but which may respond to traditional home remedies.

Surgical spirit: 'I cured my athlete's foot twenty years ago by dabbing surgical spirit between the toes. The old skin slides off, leaving lovely healthy pink skin for ever so long as you keep off the talcum. Thereafter a daily dab of cheap eau de Cologne between the toes is all that is needed.' Mrs Evelyn Woodford from Devon.

Mr G. D. Adams from Northamptonshire found that by placing the feet in a bowl of surgical spirit, 'the infection sloughed off, leaving the most beautiful pink baby skin behind with no sign of athlete's foot'. In addition, he put his socks on while his feet were still wet and sterilized his shoes by sloshing the spirit into them.

Lavender Oil: When spending the weekend at a conference, Lady Yardley from Oxford discovered that she had left behind her 'rather ineffective Boots anti-athlete's foot cream'. 'I did have some lavender oil with me which I like to use in the bath and which seemed worth trying. I was amazed to find that after a few days the persistent infection had healed completely. Cracks in the flesh were still there —but the skin was healthy.'

Saline rinse: Add two teaspoons of salt to 500 ml of hot water and soak the feet in it for ten minutes. This should be repeated daily. Salt is an antiseptic, reduces the sweatiness of the feet and softens the skin so other antifungal prescriptions can work more effectively.

Cotton wool: The importance of allowing the skin between the toes to 'breathe' is emphasized by Mr Charles Gallini from East Sussex: 'Look at your foot and see if your toes are "hermetically sealed" so the air does not get in between the toes. If that is so, the skin between the toes is not breathing and the perspiration is not drying. In other words a perfect place for germs. The solution is to separate the toes with a little cotton wool night and morning. It will not stay but as long as it does the skin will breathe.'

Antidandruff shampoo: This is a masterpiece of lateral thinking that is so obvious it is surprising it is not better known. The principle is simple: both athlete's foot and dandruff are caused by a fungus, so they should respond to the same treatment. A reader from Bath reports: 'After giving my toes a few minutes' soak in antidandruff shampoo, the dead skin almost floats away and the itching disappears. Occasional subsequent applications easily keep the condition in check.'

Mr T.I. Fowle from Kent also comments on the efficacy of this treatment: 'I first soak my feet for ten minutes or so in a solution of potassium permanganate, then soak them well with antidandruff shampoo, massaging it well between and under the toes for about a minute, rinse and dry. After doing this every day for a few weeks the cracks and redness disappeared and ever since the skin has looked and felt completely healthy. That was twenty years ago and for a long time now I have given my feet the treatment only once a week. I have used various brands of shampoo without noticing any difference.'

Back Pain

Back pain is one of the commonest of all chronic ailments because there are more muscles, nerves, bones, joints and ligaments running up the length of the spine in close proximity to each other than in any other part of the body. Further, this subtle complexity of spinal structures is such that even the best-trained doctors with the most sophisticated diagnostic equipment can find it difficult to determine the precise source of the misfortune. There are, however, three main types:

1. *Musculoskeletel backache* (otherwise known as lumbago)
   Here the pain tends to be in the muscles, joints and ligaments and comes on suddenly. The pain is likely to be worse first thing in the morning or on movement.

2. *Slipped disc backache* (otherwise known as sciatica)
   Here the pain is caused by a disc pressing on the sciatic nerve causing a sharp, shooting pain which radiates down the back of one or both legs. It often occurs after exertion or lifting and can be made worse by coughing.

3. *Inflammatory backache*
   The back pain arises from inflammation of the joints of the spine as part of a generalized inflammatory condition such as rheumatoid arthritis or ankylosing spondylitis.

There are many treatments for back pain.

Depending on the cause of the problem, they range from rest, physiotherapy and manipulation, through anti-inflammatory drugs and painkillers all the way up to a major operation. There are, however, three further home-remedy-type options that are well worth knowing about. First are various manoeuvres to lessen the risk of an attack of back pain. The second is the benefit of regular exercise to strengthen the muscles of the back, and the third is that, albeit rarely, back pain can be due to some item in the diet, and for some unknown reason lettuce is a prime offender.

PREVENTION: LESSENING THE RISK OF BACK PAIN

In bed: When lying flat, support the back by placing a cushion or pillow under the knees. This takes the pressure off the back by allowing the hamstrings to relax. Further, when getting out of bed in the morning the strain on the back can be lessened by bringing the knees up to hip level and rolling on to the side. Then the feet should be lowered on to the floor using the arms to lever yourself up in to the sitting position. A sprung mattress is a great boon.

Sitting down: When sitting, a cushion in the small of the back will lend useful support.

Those who use a keyboard regularly should keep their elbows at right angles to the desk and use a wrist rest.

Carrying, loading and lifting: Loaded shopping bags should be carried evenly, one in each hand. Handbags are probably best carried across the chest rather than over the shoulder as this can alter the mechanics of the back. Bending from the hips or stooping should be avoided, so when picking up objects or weeding the garden it is best to go down on one knee or squat.

RELIEVING THE PAIN: HEAT AND COLD

Back pain can be eased by alternating heat and cold. Two towels should be wrung out, one in hot water and one in cold. The hot towel should be applied to the affected area for three minutes and the cold towel for one minute. This process can be repeated for about twenty minutes. In the first twenty-four hours after the onset of back pain, an ice pack or bag of frozen vegetables wrapped in a clean tea towel can help to relieve inflammation in the muscles. When spasm is a major problem then a hot-water bottle wrapped in a towel and placed against the painful area often provides relief.

EXERCISE

The most effective preventive exercises for those prone to back pain are designed to stretch the lower back and strengthen the abdominal muscles.

Stretching the Lower Back: Knees-to-chest rock

Start lying on the back. Pull both knees to the chest one at a time. Hold the knees in this position. Curl head and shoulders forward and gently rock to and fro and from side to side.

Start lying on your back, *knees bent* and feet flat with the arms relaxed at your side. Then exhale and raise the upper part of the body just far enough to be able to see the navel. Hold the position and then relax. (This and several similar exercises are described in more detail in *Arthritis: What Really Works* by Dava Sobel and Arthur Klein.)

FOOD

Lettuce

Lettuce, for some inexplicable reason, can cause back pain. Mr Andrew Stronach from Kent suffered from chronic low-back pain and lumbago for ten years. He had been advised by two separate specialists that he would need to have an operation to relieve the pressure on the nerves in the spinal cords which were responsible for his symptoms. He noticed on reading *The Times* one day a reader's letter which claimed that many people had experienced lumbago as a result of eating lettuce:

As I had suffered the torture of the damned on and off for over ten years I decided to stop eating the stuff. No more pain, no more stiffness! A look back at the events of the past proved convincing. I had first had the problem while on an artillery exercise during National Service when, for some reason, we had been given lettuce every day for a fortnight—rare enough to be memorable. Since then I only suffered when living with my wife or my mother both of whom always gave me regular salads (when living on my own I never bothered).

Subsequently I have been free of pain except for those few occasions when I have succumbed to temptation and eaten lettuce. Even a leaf in a sandwich can give me the odd twinge the next day. The symptoms are definitely not psychosomatic nor am I a believer in alternative medicine. I just happened to be lucky enough to have found the cause of something that was wrecking my life. I wonder how many others are not so lucky.

Mr Stronach's observations generated a lot of interest and several people subsequently reported that they too had benefited in a similar way from a lettuce-free diet. Mr Paul Hazelwood from Warwickshire writes:

I have eaten lettuce all my life, almost every day in sandwiches. About a year ago I developed a pain in my lower back, which I put down to too much driving and bad posture. I improved my posture and did some back exercises but only really succeeded in preventing the pain from getting any worse. I thought my two weeks' summer holiday would provide some relief, as I would be doing very little driving. The pain was as sharp as ever (I was eating lettuce often twice a day during this holiday). I stopped eating lettuce the day I read the article [describing Mr Stronach's experience]. By the following evening I was feeling better and I have improved ever since.

Another female reader described a similar experience: 'With two hip replacements behind me I thought I was set up for a few years, but then both elbows began to swell with very tender bones on the inside. I could understand the years of tennis taking the right elbow but did leaning on the left one wear it away as quickly? No, it was the passion for Caesar salad with all that lettuce. Since the article describing Mr Stronach's experience, not a leaf has passed my lips and the elbows have recovered and the hips are much less stiff.'

Fruit

Several other foods can also give rise to back pain, as described by the following two readers. Mrs Sheila Dryburgh from Surrey writes: 'Many years ago I discovered the effects of eating lettuce and have not eaten it now for many years. I have a salad every day but *no lettuce*. I also found I had similar problems with citrus fruits and that eating half a grapefruit produced the startling symptoms of a slipped disc. I have never touched a grapefruit or citrus fruit since and have never had any further problems.'

Mrs Margerita Stapleton from Dorset described a similar experience with strawberries: 'Some years ago I had a crippling attack of what I thought was sciatica. I had been given several presents of strawberries to which I have always been very partial.

When the season stopped so did all my pain! Since then I have found that if I eat more than a very few, rheumatic pains follow inevitably.'

Nutmeg

Equally mysteriously, Mr J. C. Beard, a retired dentist from Watford, reports on a type of food that relieved his back pain—though this one he did not have to eat:

I am a retired dental surgeon of the 'old-fashioned school' who always stooped while operating on my patients in an orthodox dental chair. Naturally, I suffered the occasional backache until a postman patient recommended that I should keep a nutmeg in my hip pocket. Full of scepticism I tried it, and now after thirty years or so I am never without one. I mentioned this to an angling friend and to my surprise he assured me that for many years he had hung a small bag of nutmeg from his bedpost to ward off night cramps! This may be autosuggestion or witchcraft, but we agreed, as do many of my patients who tried it, that it does work for us.

Several readers with back pain were sufficiently impressed by Mr Beard's account to try nutmeg themselves, including Mr I. H. Shattock from Gwent:

Back pain has plagued me for many years

in its various forms terminating in an operation or laminectomy as it is known. Although it has meant that I can resume a normal life it does remind me from time to time that I have to stop doing whatever I shouldn't and I rest up. Having read about the nutmeg I thought I'd give it a try. Owing to the recent warm weather, or so I thought, my back was in fine fettle and during one of my frequent changes of trousers I left the ever-present nutmeg on the bedroom table. The next thing I noticed was that the gradual return of the backache was apparent. Seeing the nutmeg on the table prompted me to return it to my pocket, and lo and behold the back has resumed its normal painless state. This within a few days!

The question of why nutmeg should work in these circumstances is, of course, quite obscure, though Mrs P. Stevens from Taunton makes the following suggestion: 'Regarding the dentist and the nutmeg in his pocket, couldn't it just be that having something in his pocket (he could try a golf ball) makes him adjust his position very slightly when bending?'

Baldness

'There is one thing about baldness—it's neat.' Anon.

Balding is an almost universal and completely natural event in males. Most men view it with indifference, but for some it is the nearest thing to a catastrophe that will ever happen to them—the vast range of remedies reported over the last 2500 years reveals a consistent demand for hair restoration. Cleopatra advised the balding Julius Caesar to try a mixture of 'ground-up burnt domestic mice, horse teeth, bear grease and deer droppings'. The French recommend alcohol and beef fat, the Germans extract of bovine heart and Hungarians horseradish and mustard oil.

There is, not surprisingly, no evidence that any of these unusual 'home remedies' are the least bit effective. It has, however, been claimed that increasing the blood flow to the scalp may promote hair growth. Thus the 'popular' medical book *The Household Physician*, published at the turn of the century, advised that baldness might be prevented by 'quickening the circulation in the scalp, such as by washing the head every morning in cold water, then drying with a rough towel by vigorous rubbing and brushing with a hard brush until the scalp becomes red'. Certainly trauma to the scalp such as burns whose healing is associated with greater blood flow to the injured area is often followed by regrowth of hair at the appropriate site. Seeking to capitalize on this effect, the Japanese have reportedly developed a spiky hairbrush with which the bald purchaser is encouraged to strike the head 200 times a day (being a Japanese gadget, the number of strokes is automatically recorded).

The other obvious methods of promoting blood flow to the scalp include hanging upside down with one's legs hooked over a bar. This comes with a glowing affidavit from James Oldham, a 52-year-old sales executive from Henley and winner of the Hairgrower's Prize for 1996. 'My bald patch was reduced to a third of its original size and I regained almost half of the hair I'd lost,' he is reported as saying in *Hair Loss: The Answers* by Susan Aldridge.

Boils

When a hair follicle becomes infected by bacteria, pus forms resulting in a boil—an inflamed lump with a white centre. Boils are usually a trivial condition, which resolves once they burst, after which the skin heals. Young men, in particular, seem to be prone to multiple, painful boils—otherwise known as a

61

carbuncle—especially on the neck.

The main value of home remedies is to 'ripen' the boil by bringing it to a head by cupping or applying a poultice.

Cupping: The technique of cupping is described by Jill Nice, author of *Herbal Remedies and Home Comforts*. 'One takes a small-mouthed jar well rinsed in boiling water and as soon as is feasible without scalding the patient the mouth of the jar is placed over the boil until it cools. Suction does the rest and provided the boil is at a stage ready for treatment the core will come out neatly and without unnecessary pain.'

Hot compresses: Hot compresses are the most reliable method of bringing a boil to a head. The simplest technique is to apply cotton wool which has been dipped in hot water to which salt has been added. Pus should be cleaned away by wiping from the centre to prevent reinfection. Once all the pus has been evacuated, the area around the boil should be cleaned with hot water and patted dry with a paper towel followed by the application of some antiseptic cream.

Dock leaves: Mr Alan Grant from Devon describes his experience with dock leaves:

While serving with the RAF I contracted

four boils on the back of my neck. I was working in the medical section at the time, but conventional treatments were not working so in despair I went to the local pub to numb the pain and discomfort. A local farmworker spotted the dressing on my neck and being told I had boils, told me to apply dock leaves. Upon returning to camp I found two large dock leaves and applied them to the affected area, covered with a bandage. The following morning, I removed the bandage and there on the dock leaves were four boils completely drawn out (the fifth was a 'blind' boil which was subsequently lanced).

Poultices: Poultices to bring a boil to a head are the archetypal home remedy and, not surprisingly, there are many different forms to choose from:

Bacon fat: place a piece of bacon fat on the boil and cover it with a plaster.
Bread: mash bread together with enough hot milk to make the poultice.
Cabbages: cabbages have antiseptic and anti-inflammatory properties and can help relieve the pain of boils.
Honey: honey has antiseptic properties and is hygroscopic—it draws fluid into it helping to bring a boil to a head. Honey should be

spread over the affected area and left overnight.

Lemon: a thin slice of lemon lightly bandaged to the boil.

Oatmeal: combine oatmeal and warm water and spread the paste over a boil, cover it with gauze and a bandage and leave overnight.

Onion: apply a warm baked onion to the boil. Alternatively chop two onions and cover them with salt. Leave overnight and strain the juice. The antiseptic properties of the onion juice will help heal the boil.

Saliva: The anti-infective properties of saliva may prevent a boil developing, according to Mr Bryan Evers from West Middlesex. 'Whenever I have an incipient boil—one knows from the feel of it whether it is going to be a boil or just a spot—I apply saliva and after a couple of days it has gone. Several friends have cured their boils in the same way—very simple too.'

Breastfeeding

Hundreds of books and articles have been written about breastfeeding over the last few years. They are full of practical advice to which there is little to add other than the following observations.

The mother's diet: Maternal breast milk tastes like watered-down milk fortified with teaspoonfuls of sugar. If this oversweet liquid was the only taste experience for the newborn, one might expect them to get bored with it fairly quickly. But the flavour of breast milk varies markedly depending on the maternal diet. Many mothers report that their baby's behaviour is strongly influenced by what they themselves have had to eat. Thus the flatus-inducing properties of beans and lentils will result in both mother and child passing lots of wind. Similarly, maternal onion eating is said to cause infantile colic, spicy foods and acidic drinks lead to stomach upsets and chocolate notoriously results in diarrhoea.

Alcohol: Alcohol is held to be doubly beneficial. It increases milk production—malt beer is particularly recommended—while its appearance in breast milk is soothing and induces sleep. There is no evidence that this is harmful in moderation, though there is one account of a woman who took the 'alcohol is good for nursing mothers' rather too literally and whose consumption of fifty lagers a week produced signs of chronic alcoholism in her baby.

Cabbage leaves: Raw cabbage leaves applied

65

directly to the surface of the breast are said to reduce the physical discomfort associated with excess milk production. Their shape is peculiarly suited to this function, while their coolness is an effective antidote to the heat and soreness associated with excess milk production. There is evidence of the validity of this claim from a study conducted by doctors in South Africa who found that women who regularly applied cabbage leaves were more likely to breastfeed exclusively and do so for longer.

Sore nipples: For obvious reasons, sore nipples can be a complication of breastfeeding and for which Mrs Valerie Harnden from Devon provides the following simple remedy:

I was suffering very much from sore nipples when my youngest son was born eleven years ago and I was starting to feed him. The midwife who was coming in every day to see me suggested that three or four times a day I express a little milk, rub it round my nipples and leave them exposed for a few minutes until it had dried (she had heard on a radio programme that cows' udders were treated in this way!). The result was amazing—after two days all the soreness had disappeared and I was able to feed my son painlessly.

Broken Rib

For obvious reasons those who fall and sustain a broken rib find breathing, and particularly coughing, very painful, as movement of the rib irritates the nerve fibres around the fracture. As with all fractures this can take up to six weeks to resolve and can be complicated by lung infections because the pain on coughing makes it difficult to expectorate retained secretions.

Virtually everyone who breaks a rib will end up in casualty. There, after an X-ray has been taken to ensure that there are not associated injuries such as a collapsed lung, it is customary to send the patient on their way with some painkillers and advice that as the rib heals the pain will diminish.

At one time it was customary to strap the rib with adhesive tape, though this fell out of fashion. None the less, strapping certainly does relieve the pain, as Dr K. Norcross of Birmingham's Dudley Road Hospital observes. He analysed the records from the casualty department at Manchester Royal Infirmary before rib strapping fell out of favour: 'In 44 cases, 27 were relieved of pain by strapping, in four it was made worse and 13 gained no relief. Clearly for most patients strapping is effective in the relief of pain—if it is not it can be removed immediately.' He describes the case of one woman he treated: 'She told me she had severe pain from a fracture of the eighth rib and that before strapping was applied every breath had been very painful and she could not cough at all. Within an hour of strapping she was virtually pain-free, could breathe readily and cough and clear her chest. She was most grateful for the help that had been provided.'

Dr Norcross describes the technique as follows: 'To be effective strapping must splint the chest on the affected side, so it must be applied under moderate tension to the chest in full expiration. The strapping should cross the midline to the nipple in front and scapula at the back. In hairy men, shaving of the chest is needed first. The strapping must be inextensible (i.e., two-inch zinc oxide strapping).'

Bruises

Bruises are caused by bleeding of small blood vessels under the skin and so the most appropriate treatment is the same as for bleeding cuts—apply pressure. In the words of Marion Banyard from Suffolk: 'I remember my father getting into our car which was one of the fifties Rovers with the front door opening towards the back and the back door opening towards the front, leaving a pillar in the middle. He was getting back into the car with

68

his hand on this pillar when someone slammed the other door. He pressed his hand hard for some time as we drove on and had no bruising or swelling at all.'

Alternatively, if available, cold ice packs (or frozen vegetables from the freezer) will reduce the swelling and bruising from a bump by constricting the blood vessels under the skin, thus preventing blood and fluid leaking into the surrounding tissue. After twenty-four hours, switch to a warm compress; heat dilates the blood vessels and encourages blood flow, so the bruise disappears more quickly. Wring out a face cloth in warm water and apply to the bruise for five to ten minutes two to three times a day.

Burns

The intensity of burns are graded 'first', 'second' and 'third' degree depending on the extent of tissue damage. Second-degree burns cause immediate blistering and third-degree burns, where the skin will appear white or charred, require medical attention, so the following remedies should only be used for those with first-degree burns where the skin is reddened and painful.

For historical reasons there is often some confusion about whether the best immediate treatment for burns is cold water or some soothing oily compound such as olive oil or butter. Prior to the Second World War, cold water was believed to be dangerous for burns as being more likely to be followed by infection, and butter or olive oil were advocated instead. During the war, however, this view was turned on its head and water was found to be highly effective. The belief that oily compounds were valuable clearly persisted—a point well illustrated by Mr S.A. Skinner from Watford:

> Over sixty years ago, when I was about ten years old, holidaying on a farm during haymaking I mistakenly leaned on the tractor and put my hand (palm and fingers) on the exhaust manifold. As you can imagine, I received a very severe burn. We set off back to the farmhouse in search of the then treatment—olive oil! Unfortunately none was found and I was in such pain that I put my hand under the cold spring that flowed out of the farmhouse water supply. Each time I withdrew my hand the pain returned so I stayed there most of the afternoon. When I finally took my hand away—maybe after two or three hours—there was no more pain. There were no blisters, no scarring and no after-effects at all. My daughter subsequently became the Sister in Charge of the Regional Burns Unit and it seems

that my accidental treatment was about fifty years ahead of its time.

Cold water is the immediate first-aid remedy for burns because it reduces the pain and damage and lessens the likelihood of blisters. If possible hold the burned part of the body under cool running water for at least ten minutes, plunge it into a bucket or sink of cold water or cover it in thick cloth soaked in cold water, resoaking and reapplying the cloth as it dries out or grows warm.

Contributors have also suggested a variety of other useful agents that can be applied to ease the pain and stinging over the subsequent days until the burn has healed.

Potatoes: Potatoes are the most frequently cited of the food-based remedies for burns and can be applied raw, as potato skins or mashed: 'As a child playing at being a blacksmith, I burned my fingers badly. My mother boiled potatoes, mashed them and wrapped my hands in the mash. They soon healed without any scars,' according to Mrs Mary King from Suffolk. Similarly, a cabbage poultice can help relieve the pain, while a thin layer of honey spread on the burn and covered with a dressing promotes skin healing.

Tea: Tea, too, has its advocates and is easily applied in the form of teabags. 'Used and wet teabags should be applied, being kept moist until the pain has been reduced—being kept on for several hours if necessary. This will often prevent blistering where it would otherwise have occurred. It is, of course, the tannic acid in the tea that is effective.' Mr G.V Pride from Dorset.

Aloe vera: Aloe vera seems to be a panacea for all ills. Ms J. Orritt from Winchester reports: 'As a sufferer from multiple sclerosis with poor co-ordination, I am frequently burning or scalding myself, but since discovering aloe vera I have no fear as it is guaranteed to work.' Aloe vera may be kept as a plant in the kitchen—when all that is necessary is to break off a leaf and squeeze the moisture onto the affected skin—or alternatively it can be obtained in a gel form from most pharmacists or health food shops.

Chilblains

Chilblains are very itchy, reddish-blue swellings, usually of the hands and feet, induced by cold which restricts the circulation of blood to the extremities (to keep the core warm), thus depriving these tissues of oxygen. Chilblains have been relatively rare since the almost universal introduction of central heating but can be a serious nuisance for those with poor circulation.

The following remedies have been suggested:

Urine: 'As a child I suffered in agony from chilblains and I can still remember the pain and itching. One day when the problem was discussed with a lady visitor, she said to my mother "let her stand in her own water". Although I am now in my seventies, I can still remember that moment which banished forever the suffering of chilblains.' Anon.

Other contributors have similar comments. 'I remember an old cobbler in my village quite a few years before the last war when chamber pots were in general use. He used to say there is nothing so good for chilblains as to soak the affected part in your own water.' D. Fyrer from Yorkshire.

Soda: 'Back in the 1920s at the onset of every winter, chilblains were one of the commonest ailments in our family. The invaluable remedy was a lighted wax candle and a large piece of washing soda. The soda was held in the flame of the candle until melting and the hot liquid applied straight to the affected part. Done in the evening, it resulted in dirty sheets (the crust formed by the soda had to be left overnight) but that was a small price to pay for the relief which usually lasted the winter—or at least a major part.' T. W. Palmer from Dorset.

73

Onion: 'My chilblains would last for months each winter until I tried cutting an onion in half and rubbing the cut edge against the chilblain. Its juice soon got rid of the itching and the severity dies down.' Shirley de Ath from Hampshire.

Other home remedies from the larder include honey and egg: mix a tablespoonful of honey, glisterine and egg white in a little flour to make a paste. Spread over chilblains and leave for twenty-four hours. Alternatively, a traditional rural remedy for chilblains is to rub them with a raw potato sprinkled with salt.

Leg exercises: The poor circulation that predisposes to chilblains may be improved by leg exercises, as described by Mr John Fraser for whom chilblains were so 'irritating and painful that it was difficult to get to sleep'. His family doctor advised the following exercises: 'I laid flat on my back in bed. I then raised one leg to vertical, held it there if necessary with my hands and continuously waggled my toes for one minute. I then repeated it with the other leg. The process instantly reduced the discomfort to a point at which I got smartly off to sleep. Later I found thirty seconds per leg was sufficient.'

Choking

Choking is a potential catastrophe, and one of those emergency situations where awareness of the appropriate treatment promptly performed can be life-saving. The first imperative is to make the correct diagnosis—and particularly to distinguish choking from a heart attack. Here, luckily, there is one vital clue: the victim is silent. In addition to preventing air from getting into the lungs, the obstructing piece of food prevents air from passing over the vocal chords, which is necessary for speech. One way to recognize the emergency is to point at the dinner plate and ask 'Can you speak?' If the victim cannot, one can be sure he has food stuck in the throat—and be equally sure he will die in a few minutes unless someone acts fast. The following manoeuvres to dislodge the obstruction are recommended.

Remove the obstruction: The common initial reaction is to stick the forefinger or middle finger into the victim's throat in the hope of extracting the bolus of food. This is not a very good idea as, quite apart from the danger of having one's ·digit severely bitten, it can precipitate a spasm at the back of the throat which only makes matters worse. None the less, if the victim can be encouraged to explore the back of his own throat, it is sometimes possible to get hold of the obstructing matter—particularly if it is a large piece of meat.

Slap on the back: It is a time-honoured reaction to thump the victim vigorously on the back. This, too, is unlikely by itself to do much good, though it may stimulate a coughing fit, which can disimpact the obstruction. By contrast, backslapping may do the trick in small children if they are also held upside down to benefit from the added effects of gravity.

Raise the arms above the head: Many people attest to the efficacy of this manoeuvre. The arms should be raised 'as though trying to touch the ceiling—or the sky'. Mrs Ruth Clegg from the Isle of Anglesey reports:

> Over fifty years ago, my family was eating dinner when my mother started choking. My father tried in vain to help by slapping her back and squeezing her diaphragm. My mother was growing more desperate and we children more frightened. I was twelve at the time and suddenly remembered a snippet of information I had read somewhere. 'Shoot your right arm up,' I shouted at my mother. Willing to try anything, she complied and the pea that was causing the obstruction shot out of her mouth

and sailed across the room and hit the dining-room door ten feet away. The family burst into amazed relieved laughter and since that time 'shoot your right arm up' has been a family joke.

Bystanders can perform this manoeuvre, as Mrs Christina Thomas from Surrey describes:

My mother-in-law taught me this manoeuvre nearly forty years ago. She had trained as a nurse at the Temperance Hospital in London in the very early twenties. Only one arm is used. She always said the left one was the best but I don't know why. Facing the patient, you put his arm down at his side, grasp his wrist and briskly swing it outwards and then upwards above his head in semicircular movements. I have never known it fail. I have used it on my children, my grandchildren, an elderly lady in a club and once did it for myself. It is so wonderfully simple and effective with none of the distress occasioned by overenthusiastic thumping between the shoulder blades.

It is not clear why this arm-raising manoeuvre should work, though presumably it alters the anatomical relationship of the various structures in the back of the throat so

77

the offending item is dislodged. A similar effect can be induced by hanging from a door, as a retired nurse, Kenneth Godfrey from Nottingham, reports: 'Some sixty-five years ago I recall seeing my father choking. His condition was desperate. Backslapping had no effect at all. I remember very clearly my mother urging my father to "hold the top of the door". As his body weight was suspended by his upraised arms, the obstruction in his airway cleared.'

Heimlich's manoeuvre: The manoeuvre perfected by Henry Heimlich requires a sharp blow in the midline just underneath the diaphragm, forcing air out of the lungs under pressure. This mechanism can be simulated by inserting a cork into the mouth of an inflated balloon and squeezing it forcefully. The cork flies out, similar to the opening of a bottle of champagne.

The technique is as follows: stand behind the victim and put both arms around the waist. Make a fist with one hand and place the thumb side against the victim's abdomen just above the navel. Grasp the fist with the other hand and press it forcefully into the abdomen with a quick inward and upward thrust. Repeat five times, pausing between each thrust to see if the obstruction has been dislodged. In the twenty years since Mr Heimlich first described his manoeuvre its efficacy has been confirmed many times. Objects expelled from the throats of choking victims have included apples, hot-dogs, beef, chicken, coins, pills and sweets. One mother found her nine-month-old infant blue and lifeless in her cot and noticed that foam rubber had been gouged out of the mattress cover. A quick thrust on the baby's abdomen and the missing rubber flew out of the child's throat. There are several variants of the Heimlich's manoeuvre, as Mrs Gilda Prichett recalls happening to a friend of hers:

A fish bone had stuck in her throat. The usual tricks with bread, banging on the back etc had no effect and the rapid swelling was now blocking her windpipe. The Heimlich's manoeuvre also failed. She was drifting into unconsciousness when she heard her elderly father volunteering for a 'have a go' tracheotomy with a carving knife. Her mother, still remarkably calm considering her daughter was now blue and comatose on the dining-room floor, got hold of her by one arm and the hair and dragged her across the corridor to the bathroom where she heaved her over the edge of the bath so the edge of the tub was across her lower rib cage. She then threw her full weight at the young woman, declaring they could worry about broken ribs, punctured lungs and the like when the ambulance arrived. It worked. The fish bone was violently dislodged, daughter gradually went pink again, father had to put the carving knife back. My friend survived.

Choking alone: Dr Marilyn Dover, a social scientist from Exeter, has described the experience of choking without anyone to help her. Eating bacon and egg one evening in front of the television, 'I swallowed a morsel of food I had scarcely begun to chew . . . I was not breathing, there was not the tiniest particle of air going into or out of my windpipe,' she writes. 'I sat with what felt like a brick in my throat, relatively calmly listing my options and looking for the best solution.'

For those choking alone the Heimlich's manoeuvre is useless as it cannot be performed on oneself because hitting the abdomen is met with a reflex tightening of the abdominal muscles. Appreciating this, Dr Dover performed a variation of this manoeuvre on herself: 'I stood up, placed my clenched fist over my diaphragm [i.e., at the top of the abdomen just below the sternum], and quickly bent over double simultaneously squeezing my chest with my elbows to expel the air in my lungs.' At first nothing happened, and she tried again. This time 'the obstruction moved, it suddenly popped out of my mouth'. An alternative technique is to press the upper abdomen quickly over any firm surface such as the back of a chair or edge of a table.

Colds

Despite intensive scientific research conducted by the Medical Research Council's Common Cold Unit over many years, a cure for the cold, the most common of viral infections, has proved elusive. At one time it was hoped that the expensive antiviral compound interferon might be of value. Besides being very expensive, its potential as a remedy was finally abandoned when it was found that interferon's side effects were the same or even worse than the cold itself—including tiredness, malaise and muscular aches and pains.

There are a host of remedies that, it is claimed, will prevent a cold developing, of which the most famous, promoted by the late Nobel prize-winner Linus Pauling, is an extra-large dose of vitamin C. The following selection is, however, restricted to treatment of the main symptom—a stuffy nose.

Steam: Steam inhalation, as the cheapest and most effective of remedies, should be used much more frequently. It is much preferable to the decongestant medications procured at considerable cost from the local chemist. Boiling water is placed in a shallow pan to which a drop of menthol or eucalyptus oil may be added, and a towel is placed over the head. After fifteen minutes of steam inhalation the nostrils will be clear—at least for a while. Some people prefer to go to the bathroom, close the windows, place a towel against the door and sit on the side of the bath inhaling the steam from a really hot bath or shower. Alternatively, scatter a few drops of eucalyptus oil on a handkerchief or pillow and breathe in the vapours, which will help to unblock a stuffy nose.

Salt: Mr B. J. Fenerty from Liverpool learned the salt remedy from his grandfather who was born in 1874. One heaped teaspoon of salt is dissolved in a bottle of water and the solution placed in the hollow of the hand and snuffled up the nose. 'It always works better than the proprietary remedies prescribed by the doctor,' comments Mr Fenerty who also enclosed a letter from *The Times* pointing out that in 1919, during the height of the post-war flu epidemic, 'The only people who escaped completely were those who had used salt water constantly.'

Alcohol: Mrs Mirren Coxon passed her pre-1914 childhood in Easter Ross in the north of Scotland where they suffer from a lot of colds. 'My father took charge and stood over us while we swallowed a mug of hot toddy—whisky, honey and hot water. It cured the cold and had the bonus of putting us off whisky for life.'

Chicken soup: Chicken soup is also known as Jewish penicillin because of the long-standing belief held by Jewish mothers that it relieves infections of the upper respiratory tract. Interestingly, the dietary instructions to Moses on Mount Sinai specifically permitted chicken, and some believe the recipe for chicken soup was given to Moses on this occasion. The beneficial ingredient of the soup has recently been identified as a sulphur compound which increases the velocity of nasal secretions by almost a third, thus promoting the elimination of the infective viral particles from the nose.

Vaseline: As a cold begins to resolve, the nostril openings may be inflamed and painful from the repeated trauma of nose blowing. Vaseline (petroleum jelly) applied on a cotton-wool bud is an effective remedy, and saliva is also reputedly useful in preventing crusts and scabs forming around the nostrils.

Goose dripping: Sometimes the effect of a home remedy can be worse than the ailment for which it is intended. For Tom Chilton from Sussex, the goose dripping cure for a cold proved to be 'the very worst experience I encountered during five years in RAF Bomber Command'. He explains:

Stationed in Yorkshire in the winter of 1941 I was billeted out to the nearby village and had a stinker of a cold. The dear and very old lady I was billeted with insisted she had a lightning and infallible cure for my cold. To humour her, I allowed her to give me a large square of brown paper smothered with greasy goose dripping secured around my neck by a piece of string, this pongy mess stuck to my chest. That very day the station medical officer carried out a surprise inspection. We were all lined up, shirts off, trousers round ankles. When the medical officer reached me he couldn't believe his eyes. He gazed at the square of brown paper, he shook his head sadly, just went 'tut tut' and passed on his way. Needless to say, other airmen uttered a few more choice words. As with all colds when we are young, in three days it was gone. The old lady told all the villagers how she had cured my dreadful cold.

Cold Sores

Cold sores are caused by the herpes virus, which lurks in the nerves around the mouth. Most of the time they cause no symptoms, but periodically they track down a nerve to the surface of the skin where initially they cause a tingling sensation followed by the appearance of one or more blisters. These last several days before scabbing over. An attack may come out of the blue but more usually is precipitated by one or other of several types of stress—including a respiratory infection or exposure of the skin to cold or sunlight.

The standard medical treatment for the last ten years has been the antiviral drug Acyclovir either in the form of a cream or, for those with severe recurrent attacks, taken in the form of tablets. The doctor's bible, the *Drugs and Therapeutic Bulletin*, was not impressed by the claims of efficacy for the cream, commenting that it 'conferred no clinical advantage compared to placebos', though taking the tablets regularly does reduce the frequency of episodes. The drug is costly—at £5 for a cream and £30 for a course of tablets—so alternative remedies are of great interest.

Alcohol and spirits: Mr S. W. Sanders from Suffolk commended the aftershave lotion Tabac Original. 'This does not completely stop the cold sores but is a tremendous boon. The earlier the application, the greater and better the relief.' The active ingredient is almost certainly the alcohol base of the aftershave, as indeed must be the case with several other recommended remedies including perfumes, whisky, spirits of camphor, surgical spirit, vinegar and TCP. Dr Svant Travenius explains how alcohol works: 'The herpes virus [that causes the cold sore] needs a high humidity to be effective and capable of multiplication. If the water content in the tissues sinks below a certain minimum, the virus becomes inactivated. Alcohol is a dehydrating agent. This reduces the available water content in the sites affected by the virus, with the result that it is made ineffective and the sores heal.'

Coffee: Caffeine, the main constituent of coffee, has been shown to inhibit the herpes virus. This may account for the excellent results reported by Mr W.I. Drysdale from Devon: 'When you get that tell-tale tickle, simply dip your finger into the residue of a cup of instant black coffee and rub on the affected part. The coffee must not be decaffeinated. It need not be unnecessarily strong.' Mr Drysdale reports that fellow sufferers to whom he has commended this remedy have been equally impressed, but 'when I have mentioned it to a variety of professional people including pharmacists and doctors I have been greeted with a half-closed eye and a suggestion of a smirk'.

Earwax: Sailors are particularly prone to cold sores as the combination of sun and wind is well recognized to be a major precipitating factor, so this suggestion from Mr K. E. Smith from Gwynedd is of particular interest: 'Fifty years ago a sailor (before the mast!) suggested I use my own earwax. Distasteful maybe, but I have never had any trouble since and neither has anyone to whom I have passed on the tip.' The rationale for this remedy is presumably a mixture of the protective effect of the wax and its anti-infective properties.

Ice cube: The ice-cube remedy for piles was mentioned in the Introduction (see pages 7–8), and can also be effective in treating cold sores. The treatment involves applying the ice cubes continuously for one and a half to two hours to the incipient site of a cold sore within twenty-four hours of the first symptoms. 'The initial symptoms and pain cease immediately and healing is complete within one or two days,' reported Dr Sanford Danziger of the Hebrew University in Jerusalem in the *Lancet*. Dr David Zimmerman subsequently publicized this remedy in the *Ladies Home Journal* —a monthly US women's magazine with a circulation of six million. 'Over the next few months twenty-six readers wrote to say that they or a family member had tried the ice treatment for one or more cold sores. All said the method worked dramatically.' Comments included the following: 'For me a cold sore used to mean at least a week of pain and unsightly sores . . . when I felt a cold sore starting . . . I put ice on it for two hours. The next morning, to my delight, the blisters were gone' and 'as soon as I felt the familiar tingling of an erupting cold sore, I applied an ice cube to my lip . . . By the next morning the blister was completely gone.'

Vaseline: The opportunity to prevent cold sores emerging is limited, but as just noted, exposure to the elements is a frequent precipitant. Those prone to recurrent attacks should, when outdoors or on the beach on holiday, make sure they cover their lips with generous doses of Vaseline (petroleum jelly).

Conjunctivitis

Conjunctivitis, otherwise known as pink eye, can be caused by an infection (where there will be a greenish discharge or crusting of the eyelids in the morning), by an allergy (most usually hay fever when itching is a prominent symptom), or by an irritant such as chillies.

INFECTIVE CONJUNCTIVITIS

The standard treatment for infective conjunctivitis is an antibiotic cream or eye drops, but many cases will clear with simple hygienic measures.

Warm water compresses: Dip a flannel in warm water and apply it to the eye three or four times a day for ten minutes. In addition, a cotton-wool bud dipped in a bowl of warm water with a couple of drops of baby shampoo can be used to clear away the crusts from the eyelids.

Apple juice: Apple juice is recommended for blepharitis—infection of the eyelids—which may be associated with conjunctivitis or come on its own. 'Peel off a two-inch slice of apple, bend in half with the skin sides together until the juice appears, then place gently on the eyelids. The redness goes and so does the pus—not completely but it is kept in check if done several times a day.' Yvonne Wilson from London.

A swim: Chlorine is a very effective anti-infective agent, which is why it is added to swimming pools. A reader reports:

In the days when I wore contact lenses I was less than perfect about keeping them sterile and consequently got conjunctivitis often. I had to put up with it until I could get an appointment with the doctor, pay a prescription charge at the chemist and the drops hurt when I used them. Then one day I reflected that chlorine was put

89

in swimming pools to kill bacteria and the chlorine vapour just above the water was pretty dense. I took myself off for a swim. Ten minutes in the pool did the trick instantly, and I found there was no need to put my head under water.

Salt also has anti-infective properties, so for those living beside the sea it is possible that a quick dip in the ocean may prove equally efficacious.

Urine: Urine may seem an unlikely home remedy for conjunctivitis, but urine eye drops are a particularly appropriate way of making use of its anti-infective properties. 'Applying a few drops of fresh or boiled urine can be very helpful in cases of conjunctivitis. It is sometimes wise to dilute the urine used for eyedrops with a bit of water.' Coen van der Kroon, *The Complete Guide to Urine Therapy.*

ALLERGIC CONJUNCTIVITIS

The best treatment is undoubtedly the anti-allergic compounds Opticrom or Predsol, but warm water compresses as described for infective conjunctivitis can help relieve the symptoms of grittiness and itchiness.

90

Inadvertently rubbing the eye after having handled a chilli can cause exquisite pain and copious tears. Dr Richard Roberts, a genetic specialist in Texas and self-confessed chilli addict, describes the following interesting remedies: 'I once experienced these symptoms when in the company of several Mexican friends who urged me to put hair in the affected eye immediately. Though incredulous I grabbed for my wife's hair [his own was too short for the purpose] and the pain and tears cleared immediately. I cannot explain this effect.'

The watering eyes associated with chopping onions is another form of irritative conjunctivitis. The 'surprising solution', as commented on in the *New Scientist*, is 'to trickle cold tap water onto the wrists for a few seconds as soon as the discomfort is felt'.

Constipation

Constipation is among the commonest and curiously the most debilitating of simple ailments, being often associated with a generalized sense of lethargy and melancholy. The pursuit of regularity, therefore, besides relieving the abdominal discomfort and colicky pains, has a noticeably euphoric effect. The reason is not clear. There is no doubt that a good 'bowel action' is satisfactory primarily due to the sense of evacuation but also because the anus is richly supplied with nerve fibres which are stimulated when the bowel opens, resulting in a most pleasing sensation. Further, the internal cleansing of the bowel with enemas or colonic irrigation is reputedly very pleasurable. The British journalist Ysenda Maxton-Graham described it as 'the most satisfying loo-going experience of my life. Years of stored-up wind and matter such as old pips, stones and undigested pills are dispensed with—it is a joy to say goodbye to them.'

The colon is in a state of constant movement as contractions of the muscles in the wall impel the contents forwards. During an attack of constipation the colon is relatively inert and the traditional remedies are 'stimulant' laxatives. Mr Allan Wilson from Perthshire, who practised as a pharmacist in Selkirk in the 1930s, recalls: 'I am seventy-eight. As a teenager my mother would place two or three senna pods in half a cup of water, leaving them to soak overnight and then drinking the water in the morning convinced this "infusion" kept her regular. About the same time, my grandfather, then in his eighties, described taking a dose of extract of cascara sagrada liquid. It seemed to work for him. My aunt, with whom I resided at the time, also thought it good for me but I found it absolutely horrid to take, with an aftertaste that lasted for hours.'

These stimulant laxatives, such as senna and Epsom salts, have fallen out of fashion in recent years. Prolonged use is now recognized to cause the bowels to become dependent and indeed may lead to permanent damage.

The alternative approach, and this really only applies to those who are chronically constipated, is to improve the regularity of the bowel by 'exercising' it. The presence of faecal matter in the colon encourages the colonic contractions, so the more faecal matter that is present the greater the amount of exercise and thus the stronger, and 'fitter', the bowel becomes.

As the two major constituents of faecal matter are water and indigestible cellulose or 'fibre', then the simplest of home remedies is to increase the amount consumed.

WATER

The water content of the stool is reabsorbed as it passes down the colon, thus the higher the water intake, the less that needs to be reabsorbed and the larger the bulk of the stool. Mrs Barbara Willett from Cornwall reports: 'I became very constipated when pregnant with my first child in 1956. My family

93

doctor advised "on waking in the morning, drink half to a pint of warm water and then lie on your right side for about twenty minutes". This has worked for me all my life—I do not necessarily remain on my right side but I always drink the water. I am seventy-five now and continue to find it infallible. Many of my friends have benefited from this advice.'

The temperature of the water, another correspondent pointed out, is important as 'neither cold nor hot water works. It has to be lukewarm.' Mrs Louisa Dawson from Gloucestershire suggests a variant of this remedy: 'Cabbage water in which a cabbage has been boiled for ten to fifteen minutes.' It is, she says, 'quite pleasant with just salt and pepper—but if desired add a little Marmite or Bovril'. The alternative to warm water first thing in the morning is to drink less tea and coffee. Both are natural diuretics, increasing the quantity of urine that is passed which is dehydrating. This increases the amount of water that needs to be reabsorbed from the stool, which in turn decreases its quantity. Ms P. Austin from Middlesex writes: 'I cut down on tea and coffee gradually and increased my intake of plain water until the problem went away. Now, so long as I drink more plain water than tea and coffee every day I am not constipated.'

There is no doubt that increasing the bulk of the stool promotes its passage down the colon. This was convincingly shown in experiments conducted by Dr Denis Burkitt who compared the speed with which marker pellets were eliminated in a group of English schoolboys on a typical school diet with a similar number of Africans consuming plants and cereals all rich in 'dietary fibre'. The average African stool weighed between 300 and 500 grams and took thirty-six hours to pass, compared to that of the schoolboys which weighed between 100 and 150 grams and took twice as long to pass down the colon.

There is nothing intrinsically desirable in passing a large stool, especially if it requires consuming a rather dismal 'African-style' diet. None the less, as is now well known, many (if not all) of those with constipation do benefit from increasing the amount of fibre in their diet by increasing the quantity of fruit and vegetables consumed, and by eating bran-based cereals and wholemeal bread. This must, however, be accompanied by an increase in fluid intake, as one reader discovered only by accident. 'I have always had Allbran for breakfast, but it has never really solved the problem of constipation. However, a few months ago I drank a glass of water immediately after the Allbran and that had the desired effect. I have continued ever since and the constipation problem has been totally overcome. This is the cheapest and easiest way to overcome a health problem I have found.' It is important to recognize, however, that this 'high fibre' diet is not suitable for everyone and can cause flatulence, abdominal distension and colicky pains.

NATURAL LAXATIVES

Prunes: The laxative property of prunes has been recognized for a long time; they were described by the first radio doctor, Charles Hill, as 'nature's little workers'. Following intensive research conducted by Dr Sidney Masri of the United States Department of Agriculture, the active ingredient was identified as the chemical magnesium. In her book *The Food Pharmacy*, Jean Carper notes that 'when researchers removed the magnesium phosphate from prunes, the fruit's laxative properties dropped to zero but when they fed the powerful prune magnesium alone to mice not much happened either. It seems the famous prune chemical works only when it is in the prunes.' Those unaccustomed to eating prunes may initially experience symptoms similar to those experienced with a high-fibre diet—flatulence and abdominal distension—but the intestinal tract usually adapts within a few weeks.

Sugar: Sugar attracts water and thus generates a loose stool. Babies with constipation respond well to bottled water to which a spoonful of brown sugar has been added. In adults honey has been shown to have a similar effect.

Beer: Beer drinkers do not suffer from constipation, probably because beer combines both a high fluid intake and the laxative properties of the sugars of fermented alcohol.

Squatting: It is alleged that the lower incidence of constipation and bowel disease in Africa and Asia is not just related to a high-fibre diet producing a bulky stool but also to the widespread practice—in the absence of Western-style toilets—of squatting which facilitates the passage of the stool. A former 'old salt', Mr E. Palmer from Cornwall, recalls how this observation was put to practical use in the Navy during the last war:

In 1942 the Senior Medical Officer of the Home Fleet flagship, HMS *Duke of York*, decided that something could and should be done about the high incidence of bowel and stomach disorders in the crew. He bought a sack of bran and had it mixed into the flour used in the ship's bakery. The higher fibre content of the diet had the effect of the African diet, producing bulky loose stools and less constipation. His studies also led him to suspect that an upright sitting position when defecating was not ideal. He had the shipwrights fit wooden gratings about two inches high around the bases of the lavatory bowls, so raising the user's feet and inducing a semi-squatting position. These measures were so successful that they were introduced into all the Royal Navy's ships.

OTHER FOODS

Some people find that one particular food, though not generally recognized as having laxative properties, none the less works for them. These include:

Cashew nuts: In the words of Mrs Irene Evans from West Glamorgan:

I have been constipated all my life, but at a rather boring cocktail party I sat near a small table on which was a saucer of cashew nuts. With nothing better to do I absent-mindedly nibbled a few. I have been constipated all my life, but next morning I had a beautiful easy motion. This was such a luxurious surprise that I tried to pin down the cause and decided it must have been the cashew nuts. I now take a small handful (ten to twelve) every day just before lunch. I have never looked back, and I adore cashew nuts anyway.

Chocolate: 'My mother, who lived to be ninety-nine, never travelled without a supply of Cadbury's Bournville chocolate—her cure for constipation.' Mrs David Hilton from Kent.

Aloe vera: 'After suffering from constipation for nearly forty years I have tried enormous quantities of fruit, vegetables, water and fibre to no avail. I then read about aloe vera—the nineties wonder cure. Half a small liqueur glass either on rising or last thing at night works wonders. It bulks out the stool and gives an easy motion twice a day.' Anon.

In addition Mrs P. Whetton from Lincoln recommends five to six slices of beetroot twice a week, and Mrs Kathleen Macdonald finds extra-strong peppermint capsules—one or two a day—before meals 'excellent for constipation'.

MASSAGE

Mr Michael Keef from Herefordshire writes: 'Find a good physiotherapist and get him or her to give a course of stomach massage. My late wife was cured from chronic constipation over a period of six months with a massage once a fortnight. This is better than all the other remedies.'

Coughs

There are three main causes of a chronic persistent dry cough (i.e., one that is not due to an infection such as bronchitis or pneumonia). The cough may be allergic (as in asthma), following a viral infection (such as whooping cough) or associated with heartburn, when the acid contents of the stomach tip over into the airways. Each type of cough has its most appropriate remedies, which are therefore dealt with separately below. There is some overlap with the remedies for a cold (see page 81) and readers are referred to that section where appropriate.

GENERAL

Steam: Steam is a useful expectorant as well as soothing to the irritated airways (see Colds, pages 81–2).

Hot drink: Hot drinks that can soothe a chronic cough include honey and lemon, black tea with honey to taste, and warm milk mixed with two teaspoons of butter.

Cough medicine: Mr Norman Gardiner from Chelsea recalls this home-made cough syrup from the 'Hungry Thirties': 'Sliced swede was layered with brown sugar and placed between two plates in a warm place near the kitchen range. The juice exuded was used as a cough syrup.' In a variant of this recipe onion is substituted for the swede.

ALLERGIC

A nocturnal cough, especially if accompanied by coughing after exercise, is often a sign of mild asthma, which responds to appropriate anti-asthma medication. There was at one time a great vogue for trying to reduce exposure to the presumed allergen, such as the house dust mite, by obsessive vacuuming of the mattress and bedroom. Though theoretically sensible, the benefits of this approach are scarcely worth the extra housework involved. The chronic asthmatic cough can also be exacerbated by cold or dry air, hence the following three remedies.

Wet towels: Mrs Bolt from Yorkshire suggests that central heating may, by drying the air, cause chronic nocturnal coughs in children: 'A wet towel over the radiator or a bowl of water brings immediate relief,' she writes.

A handkerchief: Cold air can irritate the airways, resulting in a chronic cough at night for those who sleep in cold bedrooms. Mrs J. Barton from Sussex reports discovering the following remedy: 'As I coughed only at night for two winters, I thought that if I could breathe warm air at night it would help. I put my head under the bedclothes and the coughing stopped—but began again when I came up for air. The next night I put a large thin handkerchief over my whole face and breathed in and out deeply through the mouth. I think the warm air breathed out slightly warmed the cold air going in.'

There is a further form of often convulsive chronic coughing induced by an allergy, most often to aspirin, which is described in the section on sneezing (see page 225).

POST-VIRAL BRONCHITIS

The irritation of the airways may persist for several weeks following an episode of viral bronchitis such as whooping cough, resulting in a chronic persistent cough. The most popular home remedy in such circumstances is, paradoxically enough, exposure to noxious fumes.

Noxious fumes: Noxious fumes were a common treatment for the persistent cough of whooping cough in childhood. Particularly favoured were the smells from gasworks, the smoke from a steam engine and liquid tar. 'When I was a little girl at infant school about seventy years ago and I contracted whooping cough, it was thought desirable for a child to inhale the sulphurous fumes coming from the local gasworks. I was daily taken for a walk past Chelmsford gasworks and instructed to inhale deeply. It certainly did the trick.' Miss I. E. Woolford from Chelmsford.

The gasworks remedy did not work for Mrs Elizabeth Jones from Dorset, so her father resorted to more drastic measures: 'This necessitated a train journey through the Severn Tunnel. As soon as the train entered the tunnel my father opened the window and thrust my head out facing the engine. I have often thought that had a train been passing in the opposite direction, my cough might have been silenced permanently.'

Mr K. J. Thomas and his brother had a similar experience as children growing up in the coal-mining area of Glamorgan.

We both had whooping cough—about 1930—and to speed up recovery we were taken on a short railway journey which included a return trip through one of the local railway tunnels. We took deep breaths with our heads out of the window. It must have helped my brother, but I was not so fortunate and on the following weekend I was taken by my father to the coal mine where he was employed. Here I was taken into a small dark building alongside the main ventilation 'fan' for the colliery which drew up all the foul air from the mine and it was more deep breaths! Maybe this worked in my case as there were no more drastic treatments.

Tar: The fumes from liquid tar would have worked in a similar way to those from gas or coal, as this anonymous contributor points out: 'When I was young in the thirties in a North London suburb, the recognized palliative for a cough was to locate an area where street resurfacing was taking place. I have clear memories of being daily walked up and down past the roadside brazier where a cauldron of tar was being prepared and required to deeply inhale the coal tar fumes.'

Mr H. Dickinson from Lancashire adds: 'Many years ago it was a well-known fact in our area that the men who worked on the tar boiler pouring hot tar onto the road were said to never suffer from a cold. Mothers with young babies or toddlers suffering from chest colds would, when the boiler was in the area, run out and hold the child over the boiler into the thick of the fumes. This was known as "cutting the phlegm".'

Garlic: Mr G.V.S. Bucknall from Wiltshire reports this interesting home remedy from his time as a small boy at a preparatory school in Dorset during the First World War:

There was an epidemic of whooping cough at the school, and on the advice of a parent who was a Harley Street specialist we were issued with thin socks into which bits of garlic were put and which we wore inside our normal woollen stockings. The epidemic duly came to an end, whether or not as a result of the garlic, but I can't imagine what it must have been like for the staff to be surrounded by sixty or so small boys with feet reeking of garlic or for the dormitory maids who had to make our beds since we wore our garlic socks at night as well as during the day.

ACID REFLUX

The reflux of the acidic secretions of the stomach, besides causing heartburn, can also result in a chronic cough by tipping over into the airways to irritate the lungs. Here, too, a simple remedy is appropriate, as recommended by Dr Paul Glasziou to a 66-year-old woman, Mrs V, who had been coughing for twenty years. The solution is bricks, two of which are placed on either side of the top end of the bed sufficient to elevate it about 6 inches. With Mrs V now lying in bed at night at a slight incline, rather than horizontal, her acidic secretions were prevented from entering the lungs with the result that 'the cough settled and six months later had not returned'.

Cuts

There is only one immediate remedy for a bleeding cut and that is to apply pressure either by placing a clean handkerchief or tissue over the cut or, if it is long, by pushing the sides together between the thumbs of both hands. Cobwebs are reputed to stop bleeding, but this is a diversion and anyhow they are difficult to find in sufficient quantities to be of any use. If, after half an hour, the bleeding persists, a tight bandage should be applied and medical attention should be sought urgently. Once the bleeding has stopped the question arises whether the cut is sufficiently wide to warrant stitching, and if there is any doubt then again a visit to the casualty department is called for. For small cuts, however, various remedies can promote rapid healing.

Soap and water: The cut should be washed and any sand or grit removed. This reduces the risk of infection and prevents the discoloration or tattooing effect when small foreign bodies are left behind.

Egg membrane: Mrs Helen Cooper from Wareham describes this interesting alternative to the modern steri-strip. 'When I was ten years old I cut my eye just below the brow on the outer side. My mother cracked open an egg, removed a piece of the white membrane from the inside of the shell, and after cleaning the wound, placed the membrane over the cut. As it dried, so it pulled the cut together and eventually the membrane became quite hard, when it was removed revealing a healed wound underneath.' (For obvious reasons this remedy should not be tried on anyone with an allergy to egg.)

Honey: Honey has potent healing properties. Mrs M.S. Geering from Hertfordshire reports: 'Cuts, especially those caused when a knife slips, are easily and quickly cured by covering them with a coat of honey, pushing the edges together and covering it with an Elastoplast. A small cut will in this way heal overnight.'

Saliva: Saliva's curative potential is particularly

appropriate for cuts and wounds. Mrs Pamela Betts from Leicestershire believes that the phrase 'kissing it better' probably comes from the instinct to lick wounds. 'Ever since my daughter was a baby, I have licked any minor cuts and abrasions she has incurred. So long as this was done within twenty minutes, the wound healed quickly without any infection.'

Dogs lick their cuts and wounds and it is possible that the healing properties of canine saliva might be even more marked than that of humans, as Mrs Gill McAnnee of Herefordshire discovered after she trod on an upturned tumbler which caused a deep cut to her foot. 'I am the sort of person who will never go to the doctor,' she says, and so she hobbled around in pain for several weeks. Then one evening as she was watching television one of her dogs started licking the wound. By the following morning a scab had formed—and by the end of the week the cut had healed.

Cystitis

Cystitis is among the commonest of infections and many women will know of the simple remedies that are included here. The main principle is to increase the fluid intake to 'flush out' the bladder and to reduce the acidity of the urine with one or other of the alkaline-type compounds available from the chemist. Persistent or recurrent attacks of cystitis require antibiotics, which will also prevent the infection spreading up to the kidneys. Some unfortunate women have recurrent episodes of cystitis which, however, are not due to an infection as bacteria are not involved and the symptoms do not respond to antibiotics. This is known as interstitial cystitis or the urethral syndrome; its cause is not known and treatment can be very difficult.

Water: Drinking two or three litres of water over twenty-four hours will increase the urine flow—it is advised that enough should be drunk to make the urine a pale yellow colour. In addition, a hot bath, for reasons that are not clear, is very effective in relieving the pain of cystitis.

Alkalis: The burning sensation of cystitis is due to the acidity of the urine. This can be neutralized by taking one and a half teaspoonfuls of bicarbonate of soda in warm water or, if preferred, soda water or one or other of the proprietary preparations available from the chemist. This should be followed twenty minutes later by drinking a pint of cold water. As a reader reports: 'I went out and immediately bought a tub of bicarbonate of soda for 20p. I have been misery-free ever since ... Should I stray from the recommended

109

path, then a spoonful of BC removes the discomfort.'

Cranberry juice: There is good evidence that cranberry juice prevents bacteria sticking to the wall of the bladder. Dr A.E. Sobota from Ohio comments: 'The potential use of cranberry juice in the treatment of urinary tract infections might be particularly beneficial in the management of those who suffer recurrent infections. Long-term preventive measures with antibiotics present several problems including toxicity, side effects and the emergence of resistant bacteria. In contrast cranberry juice is well accepted and no clinical side effects have been observed.'

For those particularly prone to recurrent infections the following two suggestions may prove useful.

Sex: Sexual intercourse encourages the passage of bacteria up the urethra to cause bladder infections, so it is probably advisable to pass urine soon after intercourse—and for the fastidious, before as well.

Diaphragms and tampons: The insertion of diaphragms and tampons up the vagina may increase the risk of cystitis. It is worth considering alternative forms of contraception, and a sanitary towel should be used instead of tampons.

Food sensitivity: Several foods have been implicated in recurrent interstitial cystitis including alcohol, tomatoes, spices, chocolate, caffeine, citrus and other foods high in acid. It can take some time to identify the culprit, but it is well worth the effort, as the experience of Mrs Sanja Porter of Woking testifies:

It took me three years to find out that the problem was acid of any kind: citrus juice, wine, brandy, vinegar, most fruits and even marmalade. The reason it took me so long was that the various items took various times to affect the bladder and various times to clear through it. For instance, it was thirty-six hours after drinking wine before it affected me and it took three days to clear through; orange juice reacted almost immediately but the effect was over within hours; vinegar came somewhere in the middle.

I took my story to my current doctor who obviously didn't believe it, and it was a great relief for me to find another sufferer at a cocktail party. Then, at least, I was able to believe I wasn't imagining fifteen years of misery (walking downstairs was uncomfortable, a car ride was awful and sex was hell!) This fellow sufferer gave me the final answer to controlling the symptoms. I already knew that the only way to get relief during a bad attack was to sit in a bath with the water as hot as I could take it, and now she was able to tell me how to carry on living after I had inadvertently eaten something I shouldn't have. The answer was to stir one spoonful of bicarbonate of soda in half a pint of water and to drink as many half-pints as possible. As soon as the mixture hit the bladder, relief ensued! Very simple and very effective.

Finally, it is important to note that vaginal inflammation in women (due for example to thrush or the drying of the tissues associated with the menopause) can also give rise to the symptoms of cystitis by irritating the tip of the urethra. Clearly treatment of the underlying condition will provide relief, though here too food sensitivity may be important. As Mrs S.M. Towell from Hampshire reports:

For years I used to get up four or five times a night, though I did not pass much urine. I also suffered from painful ulcers inside my mouth and vulva which seemed worse when we had been on a Mediterranean holiday (gorging on endless tomatoes). An American friend gave me some cranberry jelly which by tradition helped with urinary problems, and also our

Mediterranean holidays ceased. Since then I have been free of the ulcers and find that if I avoid tomatoes and eat cranberry jelly (or drink an eggcupful of cold cranberry juice at night) I sleep through the night undisturbed.

Deafness

Oscar Wilde's father, Sir William Wilde, a distinguished ear surgeon in Dublin, once observed in an epigram his son would have been proud of: 'There are only two types of deafness—one is due to earwax and is curable. The other is not due to wax [but as we now know to nerve deafness] and is not curable.' This is not strictly true, as deafness in children in particular may be due to glue ear (an accumulation of catarrh in the middle ear) and nowadays can be cured by the insertion of grommets. Further, in adults, as discussed below, a simple manoeuvre can, by opening up the Eustachian tube that connects the middle ear to the back of the throat, allow the catarrh to drain away. None the less, earwax remains overwhelmingly the commonest cause for deafness and certainly the most easily treatable.

EARWAX

Earwax is a remarkable substance with anti-infective properties which prevent bacterial and other infections taking hold in what would otherwise be a particularly suitable environment for infection, as the earhole is both dark and moist. Probably the most important home remedy is the injunction to resist the temptation to twizzle cottonbuds into the ears as this only pushes the earwax further down and makes it more difficult to retrieve subsequently.

The solution for deafness due to earwax is to remove it using the following procedures:

Olive oil: Olive oil moistens and loosens up the earwax and should be instilled in the ear for five consecutive days before an attempt is made to syringe the ear with water.

Water and syringe: There are few things quite as satisfying for a doctor as syringing out a pair of ears blocked by wax. In goes the stream of water. Out comes a brown oily glob, the deafness is miraculously cured and the pristine earhole looks clean enough to dine off. It is probably not a good idea to try this on oneself, but a Canadian physician, Dr Maurice Ernest, describes how it can be done with the help of a plastic ketchup bottle. While he was on holiday learning to windsurf, some water shifted the wax in his ear so that it became 'quite uncomfortable or worrisome, with hearing loss'. He goes on to say: 'This sort of thing spoils one's day and a lot of time is spent opening one's mouth as wide as one can in order to equalize the air pressure on both sides of the drum. On a trip to a local grocery store I saw a yellow refillable ketchup bottle of the plastic squeeze type and this seemed like a possible instrument for the job at hand. With one hand I squeezed the bottle full of warm water about two or three times, several pieces of wax were removed and my hearing returned to normal.'

CATARRH (GLUE EAR)

If there is no wax in the ear canal, then clearly the deafness must be related to the transmission of sound either through the middle ear (which is dampened down by the presence of glue or catarrh) or along the auditory nerve up to the brain. The following simple remedy for deafness due to catarrh is not widely appreciated by doctors, as became clear when an elderly gentleman consulted Dr Patricia Houlston because two weeks previously he had woken to find he was deaf in the right ear.

'I had hoped to find a plug of wax, but both canals were clear,' she reports. 'I concluded he would need specialist help and arranged an urgent referral.' This proved unnecessary, as soon afterwards her patient met an old mate of his to whom he regaled the story of his deafness. 'His friend smiled and said "Well, that sounds like catarrh to me. What you do for that is hold your nose and blow out hard to make your ears pop—do that three times and you will be cured." My patient had followed these instructions faithfully and, sure enough, cured his deafness on the spot. Delighted, he had even taken the trouble to cancel his hospital appointment.'

Diarrhoea

The self-treatment for an acute episode of diarrhoea is simple enough. The victim should drink lots of fluids and take one or other of the several antidiarrhoeal preparations, such as Imodium, readily obtained from the local chemist. It is a different matter with chronic diarrhoea, which is usually due to some underlying abnormality of the bowel such as inflammatory or irritable bowel syndrome which naturally requires specialist attention. Food sensitivity, most convincingly to the gluten components of wheat, may need to be considered.

TODDLER'S DIARRHOEA

There are many reasons for bowel upsets in infancy, but if children between one and five years of age suffer chronic and persistent diarrhoea then, according to paediatrician Dr Hans Hoekstra, by far the most frequent cause is overconsumption of fruit juice. The child usually appears healthy enough, but may be a bit short. Enquiry inevitably reveals that 'fruit juice drinks are consumed on a more or less constant basis, providing a high number of calories and diminishing the appetite'. The solution, writes Dr Hoekstra in the medical journal *Archives of Disease in Childhood*, is to establish normal patterns of eating with regular mealtimes and to increase the amount of fat in the diet. Parents, he reports, are often initially unconvinced: 'The advice seems too simple and does not fit in with their expectation of modern specialist care. However, within days, they will notice that the advice, if followed, is very effective.'

COELIAC DISEASE

The gluten component of wheat can irritate the lining of the small bowel to cause diarrhoea, poor growth and, for reasons that are not clear, may also be associated with swelling of the joints and mouth ulcers. The result is coeliac disease. This usually presents in infancy but if mild may not become apparent until early adult life, as revealed by this account from a reader in Norfolk:

At the age of fifty, I became more and more ill over a period of about six months. I suffered from aching in the backs of my hands and fingers, wrists, top of my feet and lower back. I slowly developed bowel symptoms, felt weak and ill and my hair started to look and feel a bit like the coat of a cat that has worms! When I finally had the sense to go to my doctor he said he thought I had late-onset coeliac disease and told me to eat a gluten-free diet.

For the first week I felt no different but on the eighth day I felt far less ill and just knew that a gluten-free diet was really the answer. With hindsight, I think my gluten intolerance had always been there (I was always very thin despite eating well, had a lot of wind, was pale and picked up infections easily). My reaction to gluten occurs seventeen hours to three days after eating it. The blood vessels on the backs of my hands swell and I get rheumatism slightly ahead of the bowel symptoms. The exclusion of gluten has to be absolute. I even react to tiny quantities.

The foods that more commonly cause diarrhoea in susceptible individuals are described below:

Lettuce: 'I have found that eating lettuce, even a small amount, exacerbates what I have recently had diagnosed as moderate diverticulitis and irritable bowel syndrome. My last "bout" of lettuce-induced stomach cramps/diarrhoea happened when I inadvertently ate some lettuce when it was mixed with other salad ingredients in a restaurant. I was ill for several days.' Mrs Margaret Powelling from Paignton.

Raspberries, garlic: 'Raw raspberries and raw garlic leave me doubled up with stomach pain. Cooked raspberries are not a problem but cooked garlic, although it does not give me stomach pains, has me rushing to the toilet within about two hours of eating it. After that I am fine again.' A reader from Lincoln.

Carrots: 'Until my youngest son was about sixteen he could not eat cooked carrots as they always gave him diarrhoea. He had to have a doctor's certificate at school because no one would believe him. Raw ones never affected him.' Anthea Hanscomb from Buckinghamshire.

Droopy Eyelid

Eyelids do not merely protect the eyes and keep them moist, they also act as a pumping mechanism, moving the film of tears across the eyeball towards the lachrymal duct in the corner. Thus, those with weak eyelid muscles suffer problems with lacrimation, as a reader describes: 'For the past two years my lower eyelids drooped and filled up with liquid and my eyes became sore and bloodshot.' He was referred by his family doctor to the eye department of the local hospital where he saw a young registrar who apparently claimed he could 'find nothing wrong'.

By chance the reader fell into discussion with a new neighbour who turned out to be a nurse. She suggested he fix a piece of sticking plaster to his cheek, so that it pulled the eyelid sideways and upwards. Within a couple of hours the irritation had gone.

This sort of problem comes in two forms: the eyelid may curl inwards—known as entropion—-so that the eyelashes rub against the cornea and cause scarring, or, as in the reader's case, the eyelid may droops outwards—ectropion—creating a bloodhound expression. Taping may control the symptoms in both conditions. For definitive treatment a small operation is needed.

Dry Mouth

A dry mouth due to paucity of saliva may be part of a generalized illness or a feature of 'old age'. It is a most distressing condition making eating difficult and causing chronic dental problems as saliva is so essential to oral hygiene. There are luckily several synthetic saliva preparations available from the chemist, and a former pharmacist, Mr S. Greening-Jackson from Nottinghamshire, recommends potassium iodide dispensed as mist.pot.iod.ammon.bnf. Mr Paul Goriup from East Sussex makes the following observation: first, that red wine drunk in the evening can cause dry mouth at night, and second that central heating can have a similar effect by drying up the air for which the antidote is to place a bowl of water in each room.

Two contributors submitted unusual remedies which they maintain stimulate saliva production.

String: When Mrs Gogi Younger from Manchester discovered this treatment, her doctor advised that she should patent it: 'I put a bit of thread in my mouth, usually a small bit of thickish cotton scrunched up into a small ball, and leave it in my mouth and cheek, usually changing it a few times a day. I carry my cut-off bits in my handbag at home and am never without. I have accidentally swallowed the occasional small bit of thread many times and it has done no harm. This remedy has certainly changed my life.'

Paper handkerchief: Mr M. Nichols from Kent describes his remedy as follows: 'Cut a strip off a paper handkerchief of one and a quarter inches by approximately five inches and roll it up. Place it along the front of the mouth between the teeth. Close the mouth. Gently press the paper between the teeth while using the tip of the tongue to rotate the paper. After a repeating these movements several times, the paper does seem to activate the moisture in the mouth.'

Eczema

Eczema is much the commonest of skin conditions, which in children tends to run in families, often in association with asthma and hay fever. By contrast, in adults, eczema may be due to overreaction to some chemical or other, especially if it occurs on the hand when it is known as contact dermatitis. The precise cause can be identified by patch-testing at an allergy clinic.

Childhood eczema may be exacerbated by certain foods and, if severe, specialist advice is required with a view to investigating the possible benefits of one or other exclusion diet. In its milder forms it is usually quite easy to control by adding oil-based solutions to the bath to prevent the skin from drying and the judicious use of a steroid cream.

Oatmeal: Oatmeal baths are also recommended, as suggested by Dr Denis Drury from Buckinghamshire:

My late wife trained as a nurse at the Manchester Royal, where one of the consultants always treated eczema with "oatmeal baths". Recently my nurse daughter had a neighbour whose child had bad dry eczema. The mother was persuaded to try oatmeal treatment and *mirabile dictu*, the child was clear in three days and has remained so. The method is to put a handful of oatmeal in a flannel or sock, hold under the tap and let the water run through, or dunk it in the water and squeeze it out several times. The object is to make the water milky and have no bits.

Urine: Urine contains the emollient substance urea, and in the past builders and particularly bricklayers would wash their hands in urine to prevent the occupational dermatitis associated with handling bricks and mortar. Similarly, mothers at one time would wipe their babies with their urine-soaked nappies as it was believed that this was good for the complexion. Adding a small amount of urine to the bath is a cheaper and more readily available alternative to the emollient oils purchased from the chemist.

Eye Grit

The tissues in front of the eye—the cornea—are the most sensitive anywhere in the body for the obvious reason that were they to be damaged by a foreign body this might seriously impair one's vision. The pain caused by eye grit is thus of such intensity that it requires the immediate removal of the offending object. There are a variety of methods of achieving this:

The tongue: Mr S. J. Green from Swansea recalls: 'My mother took my head in her hands, telling me to hold my head back. She then pulled up my eyelids and with her tongue licked over the ball of my eye, removing the offending piece of grit.'

Castor oil: Mrs Cynthia Castellan from Staffordshire comments: 'When the children had a sandpit, I always kept castor oil handy for floating out sand in the eyes—also a bottle of witch hazel to soothe them afterwards (diluted on damp cotton wool).'

Hair: This remedy comes from Mr Bill Annable from Nottinghamshire:

Stand in front of the patient, remove from your head a long, strong hair. If you have not got one, borrow one from your patient or someone else close by as the hair must be strong. Make a loop with the hair. Hold the loop between the thumb and forefinger of the hand you are to use. The loop should be ideally three-eighths of an inch or less sticking out from the thumb and forefinger. With the thumb of the other hand lift or lower the eyelid in question. Ask the patient to look in the direction that exposes the debris. Let the loop or hair manoeuvre or scoop the debris away. When you have done this a few times, the debris is out in seconds. The hair does not irritate the eye and the patient has no feeling that something is being poked into the eye.

Onion: 'A good way to extract something from the eye is to give the sufferer an onion to chop—the copious tears will wash it out. Even small children can manage this under supervision which is often better than having amateurs poking around in such a sensitive area.' Mrs B. King from Buckinghamshire.

Eye Strain

Eye strain is commonly due to reading in poor light or uncorrected short-sightedness in which case the solution is quite straightforward—read in a good light, visit the optician to have your eyes tested and buy a decent pair of glasses. The symptoms of eye strain have become more common in recent years due to the introduction of the VDU or computer monitor. Here the following remedies may be of help:

Close the eyes: There are many times during the working day, speaking on the telephone for example, when it is not necessary to watch the VDU screen. This provides an opportunity to rest the eyes while simultaneously bathing them in a soothing tear secretion. This can be done by simply closing the eyes. Depending on how much time is spent on the phone, this simple suggestion can result in the eyes being rested for one or two hours a day.

Salt: Mr Harry Gale from West Sussex has used this remedy 'for years every morning with very pleasing results and it is very cheap too! Boil tap water and pour one pint onto a heaped teaspoonful of common salt and stir. Allow to cool and bottle in old sterilized eyewash bottles. Bathe eyes with eyebath as usual.'

Tea: Tea is reported to be an excellent antidote for eye strain. Mrs Patricia O'Driscoll from London describes the method she favours: 'My remedy is cold or tepid tea from the bottom of a teapot, so it is really "stewed". Straining it into a bowl will filter out the tea leaves. Then bathe the eyes with it. Alternatively, soak a pad and leave it over the eyes for half an hour or so, securing it in place with a few twists of a crêpe bandage. Freshly brewed tea is not as effective, so leave it in the pot between cups for it to gather strength.' No doubt tepid teabags directly applied to the eye might have a similar effect.

Massage: It is inadvisable to rub sore, tired eyes as they will then become swollen and red and drag the surrounding skin. Two types of simple massage can, however, be very restful, as described by Jill Knight in her book *Herbal Remedies*. The first is palming: 'Press the base of the palms of the hands gently but firmly over the closed eyes and maintain pressure for several minutes.' The second is finger massage: 'Using a little fine oil and the tops of three fingers, stroke gently from the bridge of the nose out across the eyes beneath and above the brows several times. With finger and thumb pinch the nose beneath the bridge and maintain the pressure for several seconds.'

Fainting

People faint for all manner of reasons—hunger, heat, the sight of blood or shock—but the mechanism is always the same. The blood vessels dilate and the blood pressure falls, thus critically reducing the blood flow to the brain resulting in dizziness, sweating and a blackout.

The standard first aid advice for fainting is to lay the person comfortably on the ground, and raise the feet. This increases the flow of blood returning to the heart and thus the amount pumped up to the brain. Dr Bruno Simini from Lucca in Italy has suggested an alternative manoeuvre that is remarkably simple—anyone feeling he is about to faint should raise his arms above the head. The merit of the armlifting technique is that the blood from the arm then drains into the heart, increasing the volume to be pumped out and thus counteracting the effect of the falling blood pressure.

Dr Simini claimed that this was a 'simple manoeuvre hitherto not reported', but subsequently a reader from Rugby observed: 'As a callow nineteen-year-old in Suez during the crisis I was taught this method as part of an Army physical instructor's course. It seemed to be well enough known then.'

128

Foreign Bodies

The two orifices into which small children have a tendency to stuff foreign bodies—beads, sponge, crumbs, sweets and much else besides—are the nose and the ear. Such items can be difficult to remove, necessitating long hours waiting in casualty, and so it is worth trying one or two of the following manoeuvres:

The nose: The presence of a foreign body up the nose can give rise to the most unpleasant of fetid body odours. Dr Michael Farnham, a paediatrician in Miami, describes a typical case: 'For a couple of months a two-year-old child had suffered from a body odour so unpleasant that the teacher at her nursery school insisted she be removed—even the child's mother could not stand to be near her. A thorough examination of the nose disclosed a piece of bathroom sponge with the same foul odour as that coming from the child. In an hour of its removal, the body odour had disappeared.'

Dr Eugene Guazzo, an American paediatrician, has perfected a technique for removing unwanted objects from nostrils. His instructions are as follows: 'Place one's mouth over that of the child and blow gently until a degree of resistance is felt, then give one sharp exhalation. The object should pop out.' This procedure should be carried out under medical supervision as it may be unsuitable in some cases.

The ear: Foreign objects buried deep in the ear present more of a challenge. Dr Mason Thompson from Georgia describes the following procedure which may be attempted if the object can be seen under a good light: 'I have removed small, hard objects, particularly the elusive sliding plastic bead, from the canal by using glue applied to a straightened paper clip. The procedure is accomplished by merely wetting the end of the paper clip with a small amount of rapidly drying glue; the object is visualized and the moistened tip of the paper clip is then placed against it. One waits a few seconds for drying and slowly withdraws the foreign body from the canal. The sliding hard object is more easily removed by this procedure whereas the embedded object may not be.'

Again, this procedure should be attempted only under medical supervision.

The ear may also provide a comfortable home for small creatures that crawl into it at night and prove difficult to dislodge. This certainly does require a visit to the casualty department, though the question of the best method of removal is offered here as one of the more diverting medical experiments of recent times. Numerous methods have been described for removing the common cockroach from the ear canal, the most popular of which appears to be placing mineral oil in the canal and the subsequent manual removal of the creature. More recently, a local anaesthetic spray using lignocaine has been suggested as a more effective approach to the problem.

Recently a patient presented with a cockroach in both ears and it was recognized immediately that fate had granted us the opportunity for an elegant comparative trial. We placed the time-tested mineral oil in one ear canal and the cockroach succumbed after a valiant but futile struggle, though its removal required much dexterity. In the opposite ear we sprayed 2 per cent lignocaine solution. The response was immediate; the cockroach exited the canal at a convulsive speed and attempted to escape across the floor. A fleetfooted doctor promptly applied an equally time-tested remedy and killed the creature using the simple crush method.

Dr K. O'Toole from the University of Pittsburgh suggests that this small experiment 'provides further evidence to justify the use of lignocaine for the treatment of the problem that has bugged mankind throughout recorded history'.

131

Hair Problems

When a child's hair or eyelashes become plastered together with chewing gum or plasticine, the instinctive reaction is to wash it with shampoo—but to no avail. There might seem no alternative other than to cut away the matted hair. But there is chocolate.

From personal experience Dr J.H. Marks, a physician in South Africa, noticed that chewing gum dissolved in the mouth if chocolate is eaten at the same time: 'Following this lead I have repeatedly removed chewing gum from hair by rubbing in soft melted milk chocolate and allowing it to dry. After this the hair is washed well and the chocolate and the gum come away together.'

Several other gum-removing remedies have also been recommended, including peanut butter and hair lacquer: 'The propellant "freezes" the gum and after a couple of minutes it can be taken out of the hair quite easily,' reports Mr Steven Jessop from West Sussex. (This of course should not be used on eyelashes.)

For dry hair there are shelves full of conditioners available from the local chemist and there is little point in trying out alternative home remedies. There are, however, two which are sometimes used. The first is mayonnaise which can be left on the hair for up to an hour before washing out and the second is beer sprayed onto the hair after it has been shampooed and dried.

Finally, one reader, the daughter of a chemist, recalls her father's simple remedy to prevent greying of the hair: 'He used to sell steel combs which people apparently used to dip in cold tea and comb their hair to offset the advance of greyness.'

Halitosis (Bad Breath)

Halitosis is a social killer, even more so nowadays when standards of personal hygiene are so much higher thanks to better dental care and the presence of a bath in every home. People smell sweeter now, which only compounds the misfortunes of those afflicted by 'bad' breath. Those who wonder whether their breath is offensive may try this simple test. Stick the tongue out as far as possible and lick the inside of the wrist with the underside. Allow the saliva to dry, then sniff. If the smell is strong and unpleasant you are likely to have bad breath.

The standard line on halitosis is that it is due to poor dental hygiene, with the implication that it is the sufferer's fault for neglecting to brush their teeth to get rid of the detritus that accumulates around the molars.

133

This is certainly not the whole story: those who are self-conscious about their bad breath are probably more assiduous teeth-brushers than anyone else, but they are still unable to eradicate their antisocial odours and may need to take steps to sweeten the breath.

BREATH SWEETENERS

There are several breath fresheners and mouthwashes available from the chemist without prescription. The following home remedies may also be of help:

Dental paste: Make a paste by mixing bicarbonate of soda with water and spread it over the gum line with the fingers prior to brushing the teeth. The bicarbonate will clean and polish the teeth, neutralize bacteria and sweeten the breath by altering the acidity in the mouth on which bacteria thrive.

Food and drink: Chewing or drinking one of the following freshens the breath, particularly after eating garlic or onions:

> Peppermint tea
> Aniseed
> A cardamom (used extensively in Victorian times)
> A cinnamon stick

134

A clove
A coffee bean
Fennel seeds
Orange rind
Fresh parsley leaves

Most cases of bad breath will, none the less, turn out to be due to the persistent presence of bacteria and their evil-smelling products, even though it can often be difficult to locate precisely where the bacteria are hanging out. The following possibilities should be considered:

FOREIGN BODIES

Children are prone to the vilest of breath odours due to their unfortunate habit, as explained in the section on foreign bodies (see page 129), of stuffing objects such as pieces of paper or beads up the nose. These then become the focus of infection, as described by one dentist of an eleven-year-old boy who had suffered from halitosis since the age of three: 'I could hardly bear to be near him, the odour was so bad,' he writes. The ear, nose and throat surgeon to whom the boy was referred performed a thorough examination which revealed a foreign body high up in the right nostril, presumably caused by a pellet of paper being pushed up into the nose eight years previously. This was removed and 'the smell promptly disappeared, to the relief of all concerned'.

Further confirmation of this cause of bad breath comes from a lady from Stockton.

My three-year-old granddaughter had suffered from bad breath for almost a year. She then developed nose bleeds which the doctor attributed to polyps in her nose. He said that if they continued he would need to refer her to hospital for investigation. Subsequently I saw an article discussing foreign bodies as the cause of bad breath. I mentioned to my daughter-in-law that my granddaughter could have pushed something up her nostril. She was referred to the casualty department of the North Riding Ear Nose and Throat Infirmary where a piece of folded shoebox cardboard was removed from the left nostril. The smell. has now disappeared and we are all greatly relieved.

DENTAL INFECTIONS

A further potential hidden source of halitosis is an infection lurking in a restored tooth, which is only revealed when the restoration cracks and the bad odour disappears. This occurred to a 67-year-old man who had suffered from 'socially embarrassing' halitosis for several years. He brushed his teeth obsessively and used regular antiseptic mouthwashes but these apparently 'only controlled the odour for a few hours at a time'. And then his upper first molar, which had an amalgam restoration, fractured and broke off and the halitosis promptly disappeared. 'My theory is that the odour was caused by bacteria within the restoration,' observed the dentist.

GUT INFECTION

When there is no obvious source of infection in the mouth or upper airways, alternative possibilities must be considered. The most obvious is that the odour might be coming from the gut, though on theoretical grounds this is unlikely as the intense acidity of the stomach destroys 99.9 per cent of bacteria within a few seconds. The exception is a type known as *Helicobacter*, implicated in peptic ulcers, which has ingeniously adapted to survive in this most hostile of environments. There have been several reports that after a course of antibiotics to eliminate these bacteria, patients find that their breath smells sweeter.

Commonly prescribed drugs can, for reasons unknown, be a cause of bad breath. As an American physician reported: 'Several of my patients taking isosorbride dinitrate (for the treatment of angina) have complained of halitosis, which appeared with the onset of therapy, was reversible when therapy was discontinued and recurred when therapy was resumed.'

Finally, and very importantly, halitosis that develops for the first time in those who are sixty or over can be a potentially sinister early sign of malignancy in the mouth or sinuses, and requires thorough investigation to identify its cause.

Hay Fever

Hay fever is an allergic reaction to grass or tree pollen, or to mould spores. The main triggers by season are the following: from April to June, oak, plain and birch tree pollen; from May to August, grass pollen; from June to September, weed pollen (particularly nettles), and in early autumn, mould spores and decaying leaves.

The common symptoms of hay fever are a

runny and itchy nose, sneezing and an itchy, watery discharge from the eyes. There may also be a headache and sore throat. There are many effective remedies for hay fever including antihistamine tablets such as Cetirizine, anti-inflammatory eye drops and steroid nasal sprays.

Home remedies come in two forms: 'relieving the symptoms' and 'prevention'.

RELIEVING THE SYMPTOMS

Itchy eyes: Lay a cool damp facecloth over the eyes to ease the itch. Rubbing tends to make the itching worse.

Sore/runny nose: Vaseline or petroleum jelly wiped around the nostrils should stop them becoming sore.

Blocked nose: Mr Ray Bacon from Surrey advises the following remedy for those with a blocked nose: 'Put your head over a bowl of boiling hot water with two tablespoonfuls of cider vinegar in it. Cover head and bowl with a towel. Inhale through nose as much as possible. Sometimes completely effective for up to forty-eight hours or longer.'

The medical preventive measure of 'desensitization'—exposing the patient to small doses of the allergen during the winter months—is no longer recommended, but there is a do-it-yourself variant of this with honey which several readers recommend. Mr D.J. Drewry writes: 'I am a bee-keeper and organic chemist and have sold honey to customers suffering from hay fever. The "mystery ingredient" is no doubt the very same pollen grains in the honey which cause the hayfever in the first place, and indeed it is advised that sufferers should only use honey from the locality in which they live, since then the pollens will also be local.'

Mrs Sheila Woodward from Lancashire provides the details. Starting with two jars of local honey obtained within ten miles of the home, 'About January you should take one dessertspoonful of this each day, and thus build up a resistance to local pollen. I tried this with success and repeated it for three years and now only get very minor attacks of hay fever when pollen counts are extremely high. I have recommended this several times with apparent success to other sufferers.'

The beneficial effects are described by Mr R. Leppard from West Sussex:

I have suffered from hay fever for many

years and endured the itching and runny eyes and nose and the feeling of a puffy face. I have tried various medications which only reduce the discomfort, no more. However, at the start of the hay fever season last year a friend of mine said he knew a method of minimizing or even preventing hay fever. His advice was as follows: 'Purchase comb honey or trunk honey which contains a large piece of comb. Four or five weeks before the start of the hay fever season, take one spoonful of honey including a piece of the comb daily until the end of the season, it being more effective if the honey is purchased from a local apiary.' I was rather sceptical but agreed to try it, and to my surprise and delight I found that I had no symptoms apart from slightly itchy eyes for a couple of days right at the peak of the hay fever season.

Further, it would appear that honey may abort an attack of hay fever, as described by Mrs Elizabeth Atkins from Derbyshire: 'Whenever I have a sneezing fit and itchy, raging eyes, I take a spoonful of thick honey. Within minutes all has subsided.' Interestingly, she discovered this remedy by accident. 'I always used to find something sweet helpful, then one day the only sweet item I had in the house was honey, and I was amazed at its

141

almost instant effect.' Her family doctor was apparently 'surprised' bordering on the sceptical.

A final cautionary note is, however, necessary. There is always the possibility that the honey may make the hay fever symptoms worse if the sufferer is exposed to large doses of the pollen to which he or she is sensitive. If this happens, then clearly it is inadvisable to proceed with the preventive approach.

Heartburn

Heartburn is a most distressing problem. It is caused by weakness of the band of muscle that separates the stomach from the oesophagus (whose purpose is to prevent acidic secretions regurgitating back upwards). While standing up there may be no problem, but as soon as the head hits the pillow at night the corrosive acidic juices in the stomach—capable of dissolving a lump of meat in a couple of hours—surge upwards into the oesophagus causing such discomfort as to render sleep impossible.

For many, heartburn drags on for years, waxing and waning for no apparent reason. Luckily, there is now a range of treatments available over the counter from the chemist which either singly or in combination make this one of the more treatable of chronic gut problems. The treatments include antacids

142

that neutralize the acidic secretions and drugs such as Gaviscon that create a raft of viscous material floating on top of the stomach contents. Alternatively, it is possible to 'turn off' the acidic secretions with drugs such as Tagamet—better known for the treatment of ulcers. A third approach is to accelerate the emptying of the stomach contents so that there is less acid to reflux upwards using drugs like Maxolon—though this requires a doctor's prescription.

Heartburn may also be alleviated by several types of home remedy.

Bricks: Bricks (or telephone directories) placed under the head of the bedstead to a height of six inches can, by preventing the upward flow of the gastric juices, markedly reduce the severity of heartburn. Dr M. R Patterson from Hertfordshire reports that her husband found this much more efficacious than standard medical treatment and 'he was immediately free from nocturnal pains'.

Loose trousers: Dr Octavio Bessa of Stamford, Connecticut, has identified tight trousers as a cause of abdominal discomfort and heartburn. 'Tight trouser syndrome,' he reports, 'is a self-induced medical problem which interferes with the forward propulsion of the stomach contents.' The cure is a larger pair of trousers, supported if necessary by a pair of braces.

Cream: Cream has antacidic properties. 'After suffering from debilitating heartburn for many years I found that cream taken at breakfast, a tablespoonful in each of two cups of coffee, completely obviates the need to take antacids. The cream taken at breakfast is effective for twenty-four hours,' writes Mr A.C.H. Brent-Good from the Isle of Wight.

Alcohol: It is advisable to reduce alcohol intake, especially in the evening, as this relaxes the muscle between the stomach and oesophagus, resulting in heartburn. An interesting and unexplained exception is cider, or cider vinegar, which appears to have a protective effect. Mr S. Cortis from Devon reports that her husband's heartburn has been successfully treated with cider. 'He drinks a tumbler each evening with his meal and since doing so has had no problem with acidic secretion. He finds the non-fizzy type best.'

Hiatus Hernia

Every year thousands of people are baffled to be told that they have a 'hiatus hernia'. Hernias, in the public imagination, are rather fearsome things where the gut bulges out into the groin and becomes strangulated, requiring an emergency operation. Most people would

144

be forgiven for not knowing exactly where the 'hiatus' is in the body. In fact, the term hiatus is used here in its literal sense of 'gap or opening', the gap being in the diaphragm which separates the chest from the abdomen and through which the oesophagus, or gullet, connects to the stomach. A hiatus hernia, then, is a protrusion of the upper part of the stomach upwards through the diaphragm and into the chest.

In most people a hiatus hernia causes no symptoms at all, but equally in others it can give rise to a bewildering variety of different symptoms. These include heartburn (see the previous heading, page 142), an intense pain in the upper part of the abdomen, or dyspepsia, which is indigestion associated with an uncomfortable sensation of bloatedness. Underlying these disparate symptoms, the common cause lies in the reflux of acid from the stomach into the lower part of the oesophagus whose walls as a result become red and inflamed.

There is no specific remedy for a hernia other than, as may be necessary, an operation to repair the 'hiatus' and relocate the stomach back into its proper place in the abdomen. None the less, several of the symptoms, such as heartburn, can be ameliorated by home remedies as already described. Two others that merit consideration are:

Schnapps: The combination of a hiatus hernia and acid reflux can send the oesophagus into spasm with the result that no food can go down or air be belched up. David Taylor, former Professor of Medicinal Chemistry, describes this as 'very distressing' and for which he has found the following cure: 'I have had a hiatus hernia for about thirty years. It can produce various symptoms but to me the worst is an oesophageal spasm that completely prevents anything going up or down. It can last for some time, and is very distressing. It can be completely and immediately fixed by a tot of schnapps. Vodka is very good, but I imagine that any sort would do. Compared with the treatment, or lack of it, handed out by the medical profession, this ranks as a wonder of the world.'

A gulp of air: The mechanics of the stomach associated with a hiatus hernia means that whenever the pressure in the abdomen is raised, such as when straining at a stool or climbing out of the bath, acid refluxes upwards to cause heartburn. Mrs M.L. Jones has found the following solution which has the effect of causing a contrary pressure to that which is impelling the acid upwards. 'If a sufferer takes a "gulp" of air through the mouth and keeps the mouth open when, for instance, heaving oneself out of the bath, bed-making or bending, the discomfort and pain does not occur or is considerably lessened. I have practised this for years and have had very good results.'

Hiccoughs

There were, at the last count, over a hundred 'cures' for hiccoughs, ranging from sipping water to massaging the rectum. Meanwhile, the well-publicized case of a man who had been hiccoughing for six years generated 60,000 letters of advice. This profusion of remedies reflects the fact that there is no sure-fire remedy for intractable hiccoughs, though, conversely, mild attacks can be terminated by many different manoeuvres. The source of hiccoughs is the contraction of the muscles of the diaphragm—the sheet of muscle between the lungs and the chest. The contraction expels air from the lungs, but the air is then abruptly blocked by closure of the vocal cords.

There are three main groups of remedies for hiccoughs, all of which seek to eliminate the muscular contractions of the diaphragm. The first is to physically suppress the movement of the diaphragm. The second involves stimulating the uvula—the fleshy protuberance at the back of the throat that, according to Dr Janet Travel, the world expert on hiccoughs and formerly physician to President John F. Kennedy, is a main trigger point for hiccoughs. The third is to counteract the action of the nerves that supply the diaphragm and cause muscular contractions. The following list of remedies falls broadly into these three categories:

SUPPRESSING THE CONTRACTIONS OF THE DIAPHRAGM

Breath holding: Everyone knows this remedy—hold your breath and count to forty. The reason why breath holding works is not clear, though it may be that by increasing the carbon dioxide in the blood it reduces the irritability of the diaphragm muscle. The same effect can be achieved more readily by rebreathing into a paper bag.

Splint the diaphragm: Pull the knees up into the chest or just lean forwards.

Sip water: There are three variants of this. 'My mother used to make me stand, bend over a glass of water and take a few sips from the wrong (far) side of the glass. My husband is a retired GP and can't understand why it works—but it does.' Mrs Jill Mendel from Middlesex.

'Hold nose, press ear flaps to close ear canal, and drink from a cup of water—thus holding one's breath (some assistance may be required).' Mrs Evelyn Careless of Barry.

'Take a sip of water and say a word (any word) out loud. Repeat several times until the hiccoughs stop. We were taught this as children and our word was "tiger". We had a cat of that name, or maybe it was *Tiger Tim's Weekly*, a favourite children's comic.' Miss A. Powell from Herefordshire.

Swallowing: Mrs Pamela Burden from Penge writes: 'I have found this never fails. Close the mouth and then swallow three times without taking another breath. It requires two or three goes to achieve this, as the tendency is to take another breath in between or to be interrupted by another hiccough. But persist and when you finally achieve three swallows, the hiccoughs have gone.'

STIMULATE THE UVULA

There are several suggested ways of doing this, including pulling forcibly on the tongue, stroking the back of the throat with a spoon or cottonbud, or swallowing dry granulated sugar or a lemon wedge soaked in Angostura Bitters. A combination of sugar and vinegar is particularly recommended: 'Simply drip a few drops of vinegar onto a half-teaspoonful of sugar (it will dissolve the sugar and fill the spoon) and drink it. This has the additional advantage of being a great favourite with children. My brother and I were always delighted when one of us had hiccoughs as the other one was always allowed sugar and vinegar too. I have never known this remedy for hiccoughs to fail.' Mrs Margaret MacIntyre from Dundee.

NERVE STIMULATION

The nervous system that controls the diaphragm can be stimulated by compressing the eyeballs or massaging the neck or—the most unusual of hiccough remedies— massaging the rectum. Dr Francis Fesmire of the University Hospital in Cap Florida explains: 'A 27-year-old man came to the emergency department with intractable hiccoughs for seventy-two hours. Initially gagging and tongue-pulling manoeuvres were attempted, followed by eyeball compression and massaging of the side of the neck (the carotid sinus). Rectal massage with a finger was then attempted using a slow circumferential motion. The frequency of the hiccoughs immediately began to slow and terminated within thirty seconds.'

MIND OVER HICCOUGH

As a teacher, Mr Gerry Morrish from

Hertfordshire has employed this remedy with hiccoughing children for over thirty years:

> The most important thing seems to be what one says to the sufferer and how one says it. The tone needs to be authoritative with no suggestion of doubt. 'I have a sure remedy for hiccoughs. First I need to hear you hiccough.' The sufferer tries but invariably cannot produce a hiccough to order. 'Come on now, try. Try harder. You are not putting enough effort into it.' The unfortunate patient strains himself to the utmost but nothing emerges. The effort involved seems to inhibit the muscular contractions. Then finally one says decisively, 'You can't hiccough can you? There you are—you are cured. You won't hiccough again.'

Acute Indigestion

The symptoms of acute indigestion—nausea, vomiting, abdominal pains and diarrhoea—are usually due to 'a tummy bug', or food poisoning. The appropriate proprietary remedies such as antacids, antispasmodics and drugs to control diarrhoea are readily available from the local pharmacist, and possible home remedies are considered under the relevant sections dealing with these symptoms.

Some people, however, who suffer recurrent episodes of 'acute indigestion' may well be suffering from a sensitivity to one or other components of the diet, as illustrated by the following examples:

Lettuce: Mr Paul Morris from Northants reports: 'For many years I have suffered an intestinal ache after eating lettuce. The discomfort persists for hours. This has occurred almost without fail after eating the plant and most varieties of it. I know it is lettuce from the very frequent belching outbursts which are repeated over quite long periods. To confirm my suspicions I ate lettuce when on holiday in Costa Rica. I reasoned that the method of growing the plant there would have been vastly different to the chemical method employed by growers in Europe. The results were identical.'

Mrs Oenone Ferguson from Kent adds: 'I feel ill after I eat lettuce. About five hours afterwards I have acute indigestion. I find that most of the discomfort can be alleviated by sprinkling a teaspoon of sugar over any salad containing lettuce. This practice was adopted by both my father and grandfather.'

Onions: In the words of Mrs G. Dewar from Middlesex: 'Many years ago my husband discovered that onions were having quite lethal effects on his digestive system which resulted in extreme biliousness, a swollen mouth and headaches. For a long time now we have left onions out of the diet, and this can be extremely difficult when eating out when one realizes that the amount of food "laced" with onions is collosal. Looking back to his childhood, my husband realizes that onion-based soups and stews were the probable cause of many digestive discomforts which caused him sometimes to feel really ill.'

Melon: 'About twenty years ago I became very ill three times within about two hours of having eaten melon. I would love to try again but dare not take the risk. Strangely enough I remember my mother saying to me, "It's odd, but I can't eat melon." At that time I didn't think to ask her why not.' Mrs Margot Potter from London.

Chocolate: Mrs Margaret Hirst from Cambridge reports that

During a holiday in Austria my husband drank a small glass of rich Austrian chocolate liqueur. Within two hours he became very ill with continual sickness. I have never seen him so ill before. He was better after twenty-four hours and soon recovered. Our friends were unaffected, so we thought he must have had a stomach bug. Three years later on a

153

holiday in Germany, he bought a bar of German white chocolate with a layer of dark chocolate. Some weeks later we decided to have this. Once again, several hours later my husband became ill with exactly the same symptoms. Since that time he avoids anything made from chocolate from the Continent.

Peppers: 'I get abdominal pain as though the muscles have gone into spasm and feel very nauseous and unwell for several hours after eating raw peppers (capsicums). Uncooked chilli pepper is also a culprit. I thought I was unusual and was surprised to find a long acquaintance who recently told me of a similar affliction which only came to light when he had such a violent abdominal pain he called the emergency doctor. The doctor himself suggested the root of the problem.' Mrs Helen Archer from Derbyshire.

Infant Colic

Human babies cry far longer and more loudly than the offspring of any other species. Sound levels have been recorded of 117 decibels, which is only just less than that of a pneumatic drill. Compared with the other abilities of small infants, this vocal facility is exceptionally highly developed both in power and duration, and no doubt for good reasons. It is not enough for the baby to alert its parents to the need to be fed or changed, their lives have to be made sufficiently unpleasant to force them to react—and very effective it is too.

Regrettably, some infants cannot be consoled. This is the nightmare of young parents whose difficult babies cry inconsolably for hours at a time, particularly in the evenings and despite every conceivable attention. Typically the baby draws up its legs, clenches its fists and emits high-pitched screams for several minutes, stops for a while and then starts again. This is infant colic and the question of its cause has, over the years, generated an enormous number of fanciful theories: the babies are overfed or underfed, or fed the wrong things; they suffer from an allergy, or heightened muscle tones; the fault lies with the parents who 'pick the baby up too much', or 'bounce it too much after its feed'. It has even been suggested that persistent crying by the baby is a form of malingering.

The persistence of such explanations is all the more remarkable because over a decade ago Professor R.S. Illingworth from Sheffield University convincingly showed that the reason for this persistent crying in infancy was that the baby was in pain induced by intestinal spasms. Everything fits this explanation: the rhythmical paroxysms of screaming, the accompanying loud bowel sounds and the temporary cessations following the passage of wind. Convincingly, Professor Illingworth showed that the antispasmodic drug dicyclomine was 'strikingly successful' in preventing these attacks. Regrettably, this drug is no longer available to be prescribed to young babies following some poorly substantiated reports of adverse reactions, so parents must now soldier on with less effective remedies. The following have been recommended:

Spin-dryer: Placing the colicky crying baby in its carrycot on (*not* in) the spin-dryer is well recognized to have a soothing effect. The reason is not clear but the baby is presumably relaxed by the rhythmic movement of the dryer.

A spin in a car: For similar reasons as with the spin-dryer, parents find that taking the baby for a drive during a colicky attack can be remarkably effective.

Alcohol: A small dose of alcohol has been recommended, such as a teaspoonful of brandy. This presumably relaxes the smooth muscle of the gut, preventing the build-up of the wind that contributes to the colicky attack.

Sugar: Sugar has specific analgesic or painkilling properties in infants which encouraged the Norweigian paediatrician Dr

Trond Markestad to test its efficacy in infant colic. Parents were instructed to give 2 ml of 12 per cent sucrose over a period of thirty seconds while holding the crying infant in their arms. Two-thirds of infants showed a significant improvement, stopping crying immediately and staying quiet for one half to several hours.

Mrs Jean Harrison from Bedfordshire comments: 'When my first baby was born thirty-five years ago, I lived with my mother for some months. She told me to give my colicky baby sugar in boiled water from a spoon. These old remedies, so often sniffed at, really turned out to be quite effective.' Clearly it is desirable not to overdose on this remedy, as too much sugar can damage the teeth—a precaution, it seems, that was not widely observed in the past. 'My grandmother had twelve children of her own and always seemed to be looking after grandchildren and anyone else's children in need of care. I remember her using a square of material, probably three to four inches in size. She would put a couple of spoonfuls of sugar in the centre, gather the material into a ball and tie it round tightly with a piece of tape. The sugar ball was put into the baby's mouth and the end of the tape was tied to the side of the cot or pram.' Mrs Margaret Patten from Kent.

Infertility

As virtually all couples trying to have a child will have conceived within a year, it is likely that failure to do so within this time means that there is a fertility problem. The woman may not be ovulating, or there may be a physical impediment such as blocked fallopian tubes preventing the sperm reaching the egg. Alternatively, the man may have a low sperm count. Sorting out what precisely is amiss— and how to put it right—is not necessarily very complex but it does require specialist help, so there is not much that a couple can do on their own to increase the likelihood of successful conception. The following suggestions may, however, be useful.

The woman can buy a special kit from the chemist to ascertain that she is ovulating. If this is the case, then it is appropriate to ensure that intercourse takes place most frequently around the time of ovulation—in the middle of the menstrual cycle, usually two weeks after the cessation of her monthly period.

The cause of infertility on the male side—a low sperm count—is readily determined by performing a semen analysis. There may be several reasons for this, and one of them, the temperature in the scrotum, can be treated by a simple home remedy.

Cold water: A cool ambient temperature is necessary for adequate sperm production—which is why the testes are conveniently placed outside the body. Ideally, to increase sperm numbers it would be desirable to enhance this effect by keeping the testes artificially cool throughout the day. Urologists have been working on a device that might achieve this—a sort of glorified jock strap through which cold water circulates continuously. Regrettably, the prototype seems to have an insuperable design defect which results in the steady drip of icy water down the wearer's leg.

A simple alternative is to immerse the scrotum in a large cup of cold water three times a day for at least ten minutes. The result has been described by Mrs Anne Claxton from Bristol: 'My husband was told he was almost completely infertile by a fertility expert. His sperm count was 2.5 million per millilitre which was described as "grossly abnormal . . . fertility must be low if present at all". He was advised to spray his testicles for ten minutes morning and evening with cold water and to wear loose underpants. Within three months his sperm count had risen to 56 million, and I subsequently had three pregnancies in five years—two at the first attempt.'

Abstention: Frequent intercourse naturally depletes the sperm count as it does not have time to recover. Theoretically, by allowing the number of sperm to recover, relative abstention should boost the chances of successful conception. This has been confirmed by doctors of the University of California's Medical Center. Ten men were asked to produce sperm samples after periods of abstention allocated at random. Results were dramatic. An average sperm count of 60 million per millilitre soared to 130 million after a week's abstention and the total semen volume doubled to 4 millilitres. Thus it would appear that when it comes to conceiving there can be little doubt that the male can try too hard.

Insect Bites

There is a wide range of proprietary preparations available from the chemist both to prevent and to treat insect bites. In addition, Mrs E. Eardill from County Down recommends Bonjela: 'It forms a skin almost like clingfilm and stops the intense itching.' Three home remedies have also been suggested.

Toothpaste: Mrs Linda William from St Albans reports that toothpaste topically applied stops the itching: 'I was told this in Botswana and have used it ever since.'

Hot water: Mrs Geraldine Hobson from Dorset was taught this remedy by her great-grandmother. 'Hold a flannel by the ends under a very hot tap. Wring out thoroughly and then press onto the bite. It will be almost too hot to bear but, of course, do not scald yourself. Repeat if necessary. The bite will itch even more furiously as the inflammation is "drawn out" by the heat—but after this the result is miraculous. It is more effective than any lotion or potion you can buy.'

Ice cubes: A reader from Cleveland observes: 'I recently returned from holiday in New Zealand and Australia where I received some very unfriendly insect bites. Despite the use of ointments prescribed by chemists, I only found immediate and lasting relief from rubbing with an ice cube—a remedy recommended by a doctor (in private company) and endorsed by all within hearing. It is certainly a remedy I shall use in future, not forgetting to protect my fingers.'

Insomnia

It is possible to get by with very little sleep. Leonardo da Vinci, it is claimed, trained himself to take a nap for fifteen minutes every four hours, ninety minutes in total leaving the other 22.5 hours of the day to spend productively painting and inventing. Most people do need their usual seven or eight hours, however, and the lives of insomniacs who are unable to achieve this can be fairly wretched. The proprietary preparation Nytol can be obtained from chemists without prescription, and there are two types of home remedy, lettuce and sleep hygiene.

Lettuce: The juice of the wild lettuce (*Lactuca virosa*) was for many centuries used in France as a sedative and as a 'herbal' anaesthetic for minor operations. Its soporific qualities are alluded to in the opening sentence of Beatrix Potter's *The Tale of the Flopsy Bunnies*: 'It is said that the effect of eating too much lettuce is soporific. I have never felt sleepy after eating lettuces; but then I am not a rabbit. They certainly had a very soporific effect upon the Flopsy Bunnies!' Almost, as it turned out, delivering them into the hands of Mr McGregor.

A former housemaster at an approved school, Mr J. Jolly from Cheshire, describes his experience of lettuce's sleep-inducing properties on his unruly boys:

My charges, boys of the fifteen to sixteen age group, were in dormitories for about twenty boys. The morning after having had a rather difficult 'lights out' time with boys complaining about being unable to sleep, I was overheard by an elderly cook who excused herself and interrupted the conversation stating that the traditional remedy was to give them a lettuce leaf to eat.

On my next evening-duty shift I raided the pantry for the biggest lettuce leaves I could find and dished them out as required to the slow sleepers. Hey presto! It worked. Since then I have often wondered whether test-match cricketers' lunches of large salads are responsible for so many early-afternoon dismissals.'

Further evidence for the hypnotic effects of lettuce is reported by Mr Harold Smith from Wiltshire: 'Lettuce contains morphine-like opiates. The memoir of an American country doctor describing his experience with very poor hill-billy families in the Depression describes how he called on one poor family and found them all in a deep sleep in the middle of the day. He learnt from a neighbour that poor people ate large quantities of lettuce for relief from their misery!'

Sleep hygiene: Dr Colin Espie, clinical psychologist at the University of Glasgow, provides the following advice. It starts with elementary 'sleep hygiene'.

Exercise—late afternoon or early evening is best. Avoid exercise near bedtime. Fit people have better quality sleep.

Diet—snacks before bedtime should be light and fluid intake limited. Best to maintain the routine.

Caffeine—coffee, tea and 'cola' drinks contain this; intake should be moderated.

Alcohol—regular use as a hypnotic disrupts sleeping patterns. A hot milky drink is preferable.

Environment—bed and mattress should be comfortable; room temperature should be around 65°F (18°C).

Next it is necessary to establish an optimal sleeping pattern.

1 Go to bed only when you are 'sleepy tired', not by conventional habit.
2 Put the light out immediately you retire.
3 Do not read or watch television in bed.
4 If you are not asleep within twenty minutes, get out of bed and sit and relax in another room until you are 'sleepy tired' again.
5 Repeat step 4 as often as required and also if you have any long awakenings.
6 Do not nap during the day.
7 Do not take recovery sleep to

compensate for a previous bad night.
8   Follow the programme rigidly for several
    weeks to establish an efficient and
    regular pattern.

Finally, Dr Espie gives advice on overcoming the two main impediments to sleep:

Tension: Practise a relaxation routine when in bed. Concentrate on breathing, trying to breathe deeply and slowly. Tense and relax major voluntary muscle groups in turn interspersed with breathing exercises. The groups comprise arms, neck and shoulders, faces and eyes, stomach, back and legs.

Intrusive thoughts: Tell yourself that 'sleep will come when it is ready', that 'relaxing in bed is almost as good'. Try to keep your eyes open in a darkened room and as they naturally try to close tell yourself to 'resist that just for another few seconds'. This procedure 'tempts' sleep to take over. Try to ignore irrelevant ideas and thoughts. Visualize a pleasing scene or try repeating a neutral word such as 'the' every few seconds.

165

Irritable Bowel Syndrome

The large bowel is in a state of constant movement, as the muscles in its wall contract and relax impelling its contents onwards. This wave-like motion is absent in those with irritable bowel syndrome. As a result, they suffer alternately from either constipation, where the bowel is inert, or diarrhoea, where it is overactive, with colicky pains and an excess of wind. No single cause of irritable bowel syndrome (IBS) has been identified, though the severity of the symptoms can be exacerbated by certain foods, while stress is certainly a contributory factor.

As there is no single cause of IBS, so there is no single remedy. Everyone's case of IBS is different, and finding the best treatment is very much a matter of trial and error. There are many proprietary preparations from the chemist for one or other of the several symptoms—laxatives for constipation, anti-diarrhoeal drugs for diarrhoea, charcoal tablets for wind and peppermint-based products for colic.

None of the following remedies will therefore apply to everyone, but they serve to illustrate the scope of possible treatments. Two relevant symptoms, constipation and wind, are considered elsewhere in more detail (see pages 91 and 267).

Diet: There are two important aspects to the question of diet in irritable bowel syndrome. The first concerns the general advice that patients should seek to exercise their bowel with a 'high-fibre' diet—with lots of unrefined cereals, brown bread, pasta and so on, supplemented if necessary by special fibre supplements or high-fibre cereals. This increases the bulk of the stool, thus encouraging the smooth wave-like motion of the bowel while at the same time preventing constipation.

A high-fibre diet is certainly effective in some cases, but in others it may exacerbate symptoms, particularly increasing the quantities of wind in the bowel and colicky pains. Those made worse in this way should clearly try to reduce rather than increase the amount of fibrous food in their diet.

The second aspect of diet is that certain foods will either exacerbate or in some cases dramatically relieve the condition. Finding out which food affects the bowel can really only be determined by personal experience.

The main common exacerbating foods include, as already mentioned, 'high-fibre' foods like bread and cereals; flatus-inducing foods, of which the most notorious are beans but which also include cabbage, sprouts, broccoli, cauliflower and onions; dairy products where the person is intolerant to the lactose they contain; spicy foods, particularly

167

chillies; acidic foods, including oranges, grapefruits and vinegary salad dressings; coffee, which can directly influence the nerves controlling the muscles in the walls of the bowel; and lettuce again. 'I suffered for years with what the medics thought was IBS until I took myself in hand and started eliminating various foods, eventually coming to the conclusion that lettuce was the culprit. I had no more trouble until I organized a buffet party and joined in finishing up the delicious sandwiches. Guess what they had in them— lettuce! I took to my bed for a couple of days, have never touched it since and never had any recurrence.' Mrs Freda Rose from Gloucestershire.

The list of foods that individuals have found to relieve their symptoms is equally long and highly idiosyncratic. It ranges from fizzy drinks to iceberg lettuce, from chocolate to cider. As already pointed out, the only way of identifying which foods might be helpful in this way is by trial and error.

Finally, two further causes of irritable bowel have been described. Mr A. Hoath from Dorset describes how his symptoms resolved 'within four to five weeks by throwing away all aluminium cooking utensils and using stainless steel instead—on the recommendation of my family doctor'. Another reader from Yorkshire reports that her husband's irritable bowel improved when he switched from using the local water to bottled water and improved still further on purchasing a water-filter machine. Here the probable underlying cause of the IBS was sensitivity to fluoride in the water supply. Another reader comments: 'I find that when I switch to non-fluoride toothpaste and use bottled water, my cramps, bloating, diarrhoea and exhaustion disappear. If I drink tap water my symptoms return within twenty-four hours.'

Constipation: See under Constipation, page 91. In brief, the most important remedies for constipation are water (lots of it); fibre (where appropriate) and natural laxatives such as sugar (or honey), prunes and cashew nuts.

Diarrhoea: There are several dietary remedies for diarrhoea to be found in any book of herbal medicine, including rice, oats and potatoes. None is nearly as effective as the proprietary remedies obtained from the chemist which are clearly to be preferred.

Wind: See under Wind, page 267. The main points are to avoid wind-inducing foods where possible and, when gas is trapped in the gut causing distension, to try the 'Mecca position' to aid its expulsion.

Pain: The colicky pains of IBS are the symptoms that cause most distress. As with the treatment of diarrhoea, there are several home remedies including massaging the abdomen and the topical application of heat with a hot-water bottle. But, once again, the treatments from the chemist, both painkillers and antispasmodics, are much more effective and thus to be preferred.

THE CORRECT DIAGNOSIS?

The symptoms of IBS may be indistinguishable from three other conditions as described in the following accounts:

Bile salts: 'After repeated bursts of severe diarrhoea I consulted my family doctor who diagnosed IBS and prescribed anti-diarrhoea medication,' reports a reader from Northumberland:

> The bouts continued for no apparent reason and I was referred to a consultant who advised that everything in my gut was in order and therefore IBS was the likely cause. The diarrhoea continued. It was severe, painful and unpredictable. I dared not arrange social events and holidays. I read books and leaflets on IBS and tried high-fibre, low-fibre and exclusion diets and complementary medicine, all to no avail. After a further year and some one and a half stone

lighter, I was referred to a second consultant. He listened to my story and noted in particular that I had had my gall bladder removed two years earlier. He suggested I may be sensitive to bile acid and prescribed Questran twice a day with one Imodium at night. The result was instant relief. My diarrhoea has ceased and I have regained my lost weight and social life.

Wheat sensitivity: A reader from Reading observes: 'For many years I endured the symptoms of "irritable bowel", all the while believing that bread was such a fundamental in a staple diet that it must be good for everyone. However, I read by chance a recipe which suggested ground rice as a thickener for those who wanted to avoid gluten and, out of curiosity, I stopped my intake of all foods derived from cereals. The effect on my bowel function was immediate and totally beneficial. I did, on one occasion, return to eating bread and just as immediately my bowel problem recurred.'

Lactose intolerance: According to a reader from Cheshire:

Between the ages of eighteen and thirty-five I suffered from what was termed 'irritable bowel'. No matter what I tried, I could not alleviate the symptoms. Then the condition vastly improved after a two-week stay at a hotel in Spain. I analysed everything I could think of that might have made the difference while I was away. The only important factor was that I had drunk only sterilized milk, as that was all the hotel provided. I then changed to sterilized milk at home and the vast improvement continued. I now feel sad that I was so debilitated through such a long period of my life.

Itching

Itching is something of a medical mystery. It has some relationship to pain whose nerve fibres it shares, but whereas pain is useful in forcing one to withdraw from a painful stimulus, the instinctive response to an itch is to scratch—but to what end? Then there is the curious way that scratching or rubbing an itchy area not only brings relief but pleasure, so there is an urge to carry on, even though it is absolutely certain that once the relief has worn off, the itching will return with a vengeance.

There are four main types of itching. The first is that associated with some recognizable skin complaint such as athlete's foot, eczema, scabies and ringworm, for which the treatment is obviously that of the underlying condition.

Second, a generalized itching may be a response to some food or drink or to a change in physical environment. There are reports of people itching after drinking a glass of red wine, going for a run, having a hot bath, getting into bed with their spouse and even wearing elasticated knickers. Third, there may be a hidden medical cause for generalized itching. The commonest is undoubtedly a side effect of some medication the patient is taking, but both an overactive and an underactive thyroid can cause itchiness, as can anaemia due to insufficient iron, and also diabetes, all of which will be diagnosed by appropriate blood tests. Very occasionally itching may be the first symptom of Hodgkin's disease, preceding its appearance by a year or more.

The final type of itching is 'itching of unknown cause' to which the following remedies apply. This is especially common in the older age group. There are also two particularly virulent forms of itching involving the anus and the vulva known respectively as pruritus ani and pruritus vulvae.

The general principle in treating these conditions is that the skin should not be exposed to hidden chemicals, so perfumed soaps and deodorants should be avoided. The skin should be kept moist, so emollient oils can be added to the bath or applied afterwards; these are readily available from local chemists. Last, a mild steroid ointment is often helpful, and this too can be purchased over the counter without a prescription.

Water: It is commonly believed that overfrequent bathing can exacerbate generalized itchiness. This particularly applies to the itching associated with ageing otherwise known as senile pruritus, as regular hot baths further critically reduce the amount of natural oils secreted by the skin. It would certainly seem wise to bathe only in lukewarm water rather than hot, which is more likely to dry the skin out. A reader from North London who gets itchiness in the legs following a bath reports: 'My remedy is to dry myself while still standing in the bath as the water drains away. I then spray my legs with cold water from the shower-head before drying them. It certainly stops the itching and there are no side effects.'

Water may also provide blessed relief for pruritus ani, as described by a reader from Derbyshire. 'Sit in a bath of warm water just four or five inches deep. You can keep a jacket on your upper half to keep warm. Bend your knees so they are out of the water. Keeping your feet in the water, remain in the bath for seven to twelve minutes.'

Hairdryers: Dry rubbing with a towel after a bath can exacerbate itchiness, particularly of the anal and vulval regions. It is recommended that these sites should preferably be dried with

174

a hairdryer.

Gloves: Gloves worn at night will prevent damage to the skin caused by nocturnal scratching.

Clothes: Loose-fitting cotton underwear should be worn next to the skin, as man-made fibres can cause or exacerbate itchiness. A useful hint for women afflicted with pruritus vulvae is to cut the gusset out of their tights, thus improving the circulation of air to the affected region.

Antiperspirants: Excess sweating can predispose to fungal infections, one of whose symptoms invariably includes itching. By means of some ingenious lateral thinking, a reader from Cambridge came up with this useful home remedy:

> For more years than I can remember I have been troubled with itching in the groove over my coccyx for which I have always been prescribed Timodine cream (an antifungal agent) by my GP. However, this has never been very effective, and the itchiness often kept me awake at night. Some time ago it was explained to me that underarm odour was not caused by the actual perspiration but by bacteria which breed in it, the cure being an

antiperspirant which blocks the pores. It occurred to me that the same principle might apply to my itching and so I tried applying a roll-on antiperspirant after I had passed my first motion of the day. From that application on, I have never more been troubled by the accursed itching; it is completely cured.

Diet: Certain foods may exacerbate itchiness and their exclusion from the diet can bring blessed relief. It is well known that some cases of child eczema may respond dramatically to a dairy-free diet. For reasons unknown, coffee is said to be an important exacerbating factor in pruritus ani, and less convincingly beer, chocolate and tomato ketchup have been implicated in a similar way. Mr Brian Marritt from Surrey describes his experience with cheese.

About ten years ago I began to get very itchy skin especially on my arms, legs and back, and scratching caused very nasty rashes. It was considered to be dry skin and I used various creams but the irritation continued. I tried leaving various foods out of my diet and my wife changed the washing detergent to non-biological. I even blamed our affectionate cat and kept my distance for about three months! All to no avail. As a great lover of cheese, in particular a good Cheddar, I began to wonder if that was the culprit. I gave up this particular pleasure, and lo and behold! The itching and rashes gradually eased off, but eating even a small cube of cheese would start off the itching once again.

Jetlag

Few readers' remedies are quite as unusual as the suggestion from Mrs Hazel Chitty of Northumberland for a preventive measure against jetlag: 'Some years ago I heard a foreign correspondent being asked how he dealt with jetlag,' she writes. 'He said he had never suffered from it because, when travelling on an aeroplane, he always wore paper bags on his feet under his socks. He claimed it was very effective and, with the amount of travelling he had to do, he should know.'

Inspired by this, Mrs Eva Wegg from Cheshire decided to test it out with the following result: 'I confirm that putting two layers of brown paper in my shoes when travelling to Canada (through several time zones) this summer did the trick. I estimated we were awake almost twenty-four hours before our first night's sleep, yet I awoke fresh as a daisy the next morning. This happened, I may say, to someone who has been known

177

to suffer jetlag between Heathrow and Manchester!'

There is certainly a theory that a major cause of jetlag might be pooling of blood in the lower limbs, though it is difficult to see how putting paper bags on the feet would make much difference. None the less, another reader, Mrs Betty Nicol from Devon, reports that besides preventing jetlag the brown bag remedy also stopped her developing swelling of the ankles:

> My husband and I flew to Santiago de Chile from Bristol, changing in Amsterdam. The flight took twenty-three hours. I have travelled all over the world by air and have always suffered badly swollen ankles. I had read about the bag remedy and thought it worth a try. I put the brown bags bought from our local greengrocer on my feet after we left Amsterdam and on arrival in Santiago found that although my ankles were a little pudgy, there was nothing like the swelling normally experienced. I put my slippers on over the bags but you do need to take several with you as they tear easily.

Laryngitis

The time-honoured advice for the hoarseness associated with laryngitis is to recommend gargling with salt water or soluble aspirin, but whether it does much good is debatable. At one time Robert Feder, a voice specialist from Los Angeles, persuaded fifty volunteers to gargle with a radio-opaque dye while he took X-rays of their necks. These showed that the dye got nowhere near the vocal cords: as each volunteer gargled, the tongue arched up so preventing any fluid from passing into the pharynx to soothe them. The following home remedies may also be worth trying:

Raw egg: Mrs Shirley White from Plymouth writes: 'I used to sing in the church choir as a teenager and was due to sing a major solo on Easter Sunday. The previous evening I went to a party and was up till the early hours talking, reciting and telling stories. When I woke later that morning, I discovered I had completely lost my voice. My grandmother, a professional singer, suggested I crack a large egg into a cup and swallow it down whole (not beaten). This I did, albeit with some reluctance, and sure enough my voice returned and I sang my solo.'

Friar's balsam inhalation: 'Throughout my teaching life I had bouts of laryngitis and the best remedy I found was friar's balsam in boiling water in a jug and inhaled with a towel over the head. This way the vapours from the balsam reached and soothed the larynx.' Anon.

Honey: Here the advice is to drip honey down the back of the throat.

Stay silent: The professional singer Robert Tear advises that the only effective treatment for the inflamed vocal cords of laryngitis is to rest them by not talking and, above all, 'avoid speaking on the phone'.

Migraine

There is no single cause of migraine. Many different factors can be involved in controlling the size of the arteries in the brain, whose initial constriction reduces the blood-flow, causing the warning symptoms, and whose subsequent dilation produces the crashing headache. It is not at all surprising that a treatment that works miraculously for one person might be ineffective for another. The standard medical drugs are certainly effective for many. Mrs Constance Benton from London reduced her monthly 96-hour ordeal to eight hours with Imigran injections. Mrs Marjorie Wells of Bristol reports that 'after years of migraine attacks and having every tablet', she found that Cafergot suppositories—combining caffeine and ergotamine—provided 'instant relief'.

Three contributors discovered, by accident, that drugs taken for a different condition altogether combated their migraine. Mr Clive Mills from Nuneaton, who has suffered migraines for thirty years, says, 'I used to lose three days of my life at ten-day intervals.' Then he was given diltiazem for his angina and he has had no migraine attacks since. He writes that he can even 'eat chocolate and drink red wine with impunity'. Mr P Mason found that Prozac had the same effect, and Mrs Penny Bullivant of Salisbury found that the betablockers she took for her raised blood-pressure stopped her migraines immediately. In fact, betablockers are a well-recognized preventive treatment for migraine, as indeed is a small dose of daily aspirin. Dr R.M. Miller of Sussex particularly recommends aspirin as being beneficial in a major attack quite independent of its analgesic effects.

Two simple remedies suggest some relationship between stomach biliousness and migraine, where treating the former prevents the onset of the latter. Mr A.L. Baker of Dorset suggests a heaped teaspoon of Eno Fruit Salts in half a glass of water. Mrs Rosemary Stanbury of Swindon swears by the same thing in the form of two pints of soda water. She writes: 'Within ten minutes the eyes are better and the following headache is negligible.'

Mrs Marianne Ticehurst from Essex observes: 'One of my many [symptoms] was a swollen left eye and congested left nostril.' She started to use the nasal decongestant Otrivine, right at the beginning of an attack—or when she anticipated that one was on the way. She observed: 'Gradually the attacks reduced in number and now I do not have migraines at all.'

Two dentists, Mr Rory Linden-Kelly and Mr Robert Cawley, have discovered an association between migraine and increased muscle spasm around the jaw. Their treatment involves wearing an acrylic appliance over the teeth at night to prevent the subconscious grinding habit. This reduces the muscle spasm and can prevent migraine.

Despite the disparate nature of these remedies, a common theme seems to be that together with the well-known dietary precipitants of migraine, disturbances in the stomach, nasal area and teeth may also be a contributory factor. Thus treatment directed at these areas may prove effective.

Further suggestions include:

Alcohol: A hangover may be preferable to migraine, as Mrs B. Pledger from Bedfordshire reports:

If I mention this to anyone, hands are

thrown up in shock horror but it has worked wonders. My son suffered severely with migraines for many years. Just a few years back he came home from work with all the usual symptoms and felt very ill. I asked him to try half a sherry glass of whisky and within a matter of minutes almost all the migraine symptoms disappeared. I suggested he have another half-glass, and apart from a heavy head he was fine. He had to be off work for several days after a bad migraine, but with this treatment he can lead a normal life, though with a slightly heavy head next day. His migraines are very few these days.

A very hot drink: A reader reports: 'I used to get occasional mild classic migraine, the attacks lasting 24–48 hours. I discovered by chance that when the visual auras, which could be quite disabling, first started, I could stop the symptoms and abort the attack either by having a very hot drink or by lying flat on my back on the floor (no pillow). Only a few minutes were necessary. This worked practically every time and led me to carry a thermos of very hot water with me on days out. Outside home it is easier to have a drink than to create a commotion by lying flat on your back!'

Mr Alan Smith from Northampton describes a variant of this—hot, very sweet tea: 'I have suffered from migraines since 1940. In the late seventies I was an outpatient at the Royal Free Hospital where the consultant neurologist classified the migraines as "intractable". My own painkilling prescription, used as soon as a migraine starts, is a cup of hot tea with three teaspoonfuls of sugar (which I normally do not use). The rate of success is around 80–90 per cent. A godsend.'

Ice cubes: 'My husband suffers from cluster headaches which are extremely severe. He can sometimes prevent a single "migraine" developing if he applies ice to the area above the left eye which is the centre of the pain. It is important to try this before the pain has taken hold, but it works often enough to be worth a try.' Mrs Margaret McIntyre from Dundee.

Head bandage: This remedy features in Shakespeare's *Othello* when Desdemona binds her husband's head with the handkerchief that will later be her undoing:

O: I have a pain upon my forehead here.
D: Faith, that's with watching; 'twill away again. Let me but bind it hard, within this hour. It will be well.

Feverfew: Feverfew (*Tanacetum parthenium*) is a plant that has been used since the eighteenth century to prevent migraine and has been accepted as a treatment by the British

Migraine Society. It probably works by regulating the flow of blood to the brain. It is advised that people should eat two to three leaves daily, preferably in a sandwich to disguise the bitter taste. The plant can be raised from seed and is widely available from garden suppliers.

Diet: There are many dietary precipitants of migraine which, luckily, sufferers are usually quite able to identify. They include chocolate, wine and cheese. Interestingly, in view of the hot sweet tea whose curative properties are mentioned above, honey may also be a precipitant, as Mr Ken Sansom from Walsall reports: 'Many years ago my wife and I decided to have honey on our breakfast toast instead of the usual marmalade. I began to have severe headaches and it was not until later, when for some reason or other we did not have honey for about a week, that my headaches disappeared. It was only then that I made the connection. Several years later we changed our morning cereal and I started with the headaches again. When I checked what was in the cereal, I realized that the clusters of oats were stuck together with honey!'

Mouth Ulcers

The cause of mouth (or aphthous) ulcers is not known. They may be a symptom, again for reasons unknown, of the malabsorption syndrome caused by a sensitivity to the gluten component of wheat known as coeliac disease (see page 117). Mouth ulcers may be alleviated by the proprietary aspirin-based preparation Bonjela, and by a steroid-containing ointment, Adcortyl in Orabase. They may in addition predispose to a bacterial infection in the surrounding tissue for which antibiotic treatment is appropriate. The main principle of self-treatment involves cauterizing the ulcers which, though painful at the time, apparently promotes rapid healing.

Pineapple: The benefits of pineapple were reported by Mrs Doreen Briggs of Hertfordshire in the magazine *Here's Health.* 'I have suffered from mouth ulcers for over fifty years right from my teens and have had various treatments, and in the end been prescribed steroids for twenty-seven years with not really that much success.' Subsequently a friend passed on to Mrs Briggs a tip from a hospital consultant that she should try fresh pineapple. 'I said straight away that eating fresh pineapple would give me mouth ulcers, but thought I must try it. Well, I have found it amazing. After all those years of having the misery of constant mouth ulcers—sometimes as many as twelve at a time—I now hardly have them at all. The pineapple can be cut up and frozen in small quantities, and now I only eat it when I feel an ulcer coming and it soon goes.'

Other types of acidic fruits are likely to be similarly effective, including grapefruit as recommended by one reader. 'Chew the rind of a quartered fresh grapefruit, sugared if necessary. Let the juice swill around the sore spots. Repeat during the day. Painful, but it works.'

Ice cubes: 'I have found that an ice cube (placed in clingfilm) applied to mouth ulcers considerably shortens their life, and if applied at the first sign of soreness it will prevent them. This can be quite painful (which is how you know you have got the right spot!). I usually treat them about three or four times a day depending on the severity. It really does work.' Mrs M. Bolt from Gloucestershire.

Diet: It is possible that certain foods may be a specific cause of mouth ulcers in some individuals. Mr Alan Banks from Bath describes his experience with chocolate: 'My granddaughter, now aged twenty-five, had suffered from painful mouth ulcers since childhood, and she was rarely free of them. She had a great liking for chocolate and admitted that once she started on a bar or box, she could not resist overindulging. A year ago, after noticing that chewing chocolate always irritated her mouth ulcers more than other foods, she decided to stop eating it altogether. Since then, to her great relief, no more ulcers have appeared.'

Toothpaste: Mrs E. Meyer from Chorley describes this remedy she found 'quite by chance':

I had a whim to try Macleans bicarbonate of soda toothpaste and found, to my astonishment, that after using it for two months I had had no mouth ulcers during that time, and this happy state has continued ever since. Previously I have been plagued with at least one a month, often more. As soon as I realized what was happening I bought my son, who has also suffered from mouth ulcers, a tube of Macleans, with similar results. I was so delighted that I wrote to the manufacturers saying it was a pity they did not advertise this, to help many more sufferers. They replied that it would cost too much to prove clinically that this was so, and without official testing they would not be able to advertise it in this way.

Nails

There is a litany of conditions that can interfere with both finger and toe nails. Fungal infections can get underneath and loosen the nail from its bed, while every skin ailment from eczema to psoriasis can adversely affect their growth. More commonly, the nails may be either too brittle and break easily, or too soft. The clue to both conditions lies in the water content of the nail, which should be about 18 per cent. If this falls, brittleness results; if it rises, softness. This dictates the appropriate treatment.

Brittle nails: The low water content that usually accounts for brittle nails may be associated with dry skin or excessive use of nail enamel and cleaning agents which have a dehydrating effect. Treatment requires rehydrating the nails by soaking them in lukewarm water for fifteen minutes at bedtime, followed by an application of a protective moisturizer.

Soft nails: Soft nails can be hardened by an application of formalin, which according to the *New Scientist* can transform them into 'strong talons capable of ripping out drawing pins or even opening packets of teabags'. Formalin can cause allergic reactions, however, or the benefits may 'overshoot' with the result that

189

soft nails end up brittle and breakable. Split nails are a particular occupational hazard for guitarists and the favoured remedy is either superglue or Sellotape.

Nappy Rash

The bright red splash around the genital area of a young baby is quite unmistakably nappy rash. It looks more serious than it really is, and certainly babies often seem relatively undisturbed by it. None the less, parents are naturally keen that nappy rash be treated, and the obvious solution is to mitigate the circumstances that gave rise to the rash in the first place—the excoriation of the skin by a combination of dampness and poor aeration, which predisposes to a fungal infection. Hence the instinctive and correct response, which is to keep the baby out of nappies for as long as possible and apply some barrier cream to protect the skin from the dampness of a 'wet nappy'. If this is insufficient then an antifungal preparation like Timodene may do the trick. The egg remedy that follows presumably works by promoting healing of the skin. It is of special importance, however, as it highlights the admittedly rare but potentially serious side effects that can arise from home remedy treatment. Mrs Mary Chrusciel from Kent reports what happened when her grandson developed nappy rash:

The consultant at the hospital where he was born prescribed a course of the antifungal drug Nystatin and also the antifungal cream Timodene for the affected area. There was no improvement and a second course was embarked upon; meanwhile the midwife advised a barrier cream to protect the sore skin but refused to recommend any particular brand. The consultant said that there was some improvement but my daughter-in-law did not agree. In desperation she took her baby to her own family doctor. This gentleman said she could try applying white of egg to the sore area, though he could not officially recommend this due to the risk of salmonella. The white of egg is put into a cup and gently stirred (not whipped as for a meringue!) and then applied with fingers. This treatment proved to be extremely successful, the sores cleared up very quickly and the skin was healed.

The potential danger of this remedy is for babies who are allergic to eggs, as described by another mother. 'I duly applied some egg white to my eight-month-old daughter who had sore, broken skin. Within five minutes she suffered a severe allergic reaction and her entire body was covered in swellings similar to a stinging-nettle rash which greatly distressed her. Fortunately the swelling subsided and no further treatment was required, but it could have been a very different matter.'

Night Cramps

Everyone gets night cramps from time to time. If prolonged, they may propel the sufferer out of a warm bed to spend minutes walking up and down the bedroom floor. They become more frequent with the passage of years and, for those seriously afflicted, can disrupt a restful night's sleep. The pain is caused by acute spasm of the muscles and its cause is not known. Standard medical therapy is quinine sulphate tablets taken on retiring, though why it should work is again not known.

There are a variety of home remedies, including two of the most unusual in this collection—magnets and corks.

Tonic water: Tonic water contains quinine, and a tumblerful on retiring is reputed to be as effective as quinine sulphate tablets.

Pillows: Those who suffer from cramps are advised to keep their legs flexed in bed by, for example, placing a pillow under the knee or against the foot. This prevents the leg muscles from relaxing completely and thus going into spasm.

Cold tray: A lady from Essex reports that she keeps a metal tray beside her bed. 'Stepping on its ice-cold surface clears the cramp immediately.'

Exercises: Lady Ford from East Lothian suggests the following manoeuvre: 'Stand facing a wall about a yard away and place both arms flat against it. Brace legs, straighten knees and push hard ten times, then relax. Repeat two or three times.' Alternatively, Mr F.A. Murphy from Merseyside has a simpler suggestion: 'If you have cramp in the legs, point the big toe upwards and it goes.'

The preventive exercise is described by Mrs Mavis Huntington from Cumbria. 'I was telling a farmer's widow—an old lady in her mid-eighties—that in recent weeks I had been suffering from frequent attacks of cramp during the night. She immediately said, "I can tell you how to avoid that. When you get into bed, lie on your back with legs straight out and feet up at an angle of ninety degrees. Press hard down on the heels and back of the knees for a count of six. You will find that a sure cure." I must admit to being sceptical but have tried it with total success for seven nights.'

Rebreathing: Miss R.T. Clark from Newmarket

suggests a remedy similar to the 'paper bag cure' for hiccoughs (see page 148). 'At the onset of leg cramps I cup my hands closely over mouth and nose and breathe deeply, thus reinhaling the exhaled breath. Gradually, the inhaled carbon dioxide reaches the taut muscles and relaxes them. It may take forty to fifty breaths but it always works and the cramp does not return.'

Corks: Mrs M.S. Geering from Hertfordshire reports: 'Both my late husband and I used to have our sleep broken by cramps perhaps two or three times a week. When visiting my doctor on another matter I mentioned this to him and he suggested I put a cork under our mattress. This I did without telling my husband. Neither of us suffered cramp again. The first my husband knew about the cork was six months later when a dinner-party guest mentioned he suffered from cramps and I passed this remedy on to him.'

This account is particularly compelling because it would appear that the cork worked for Mrs Geering's husband even though he was unaware of its presence under the mattress. Mrs Angela Breckon from Huntingdon describes a similar instance where the remedy worked independently for both partners: 'Many years ago I was told to put a few corks beneath my mattress. It worked wonders. No more creeping out on the cold kitchen floor to alleviate it. My husband did not believe in it until his leg cramps became more frequent—when he tried it too. Complete success. The ladies from the Social Services, however, did wonder whether the corks might have had something to do with secret drinking.'

If the cork is displaced for any reason, the remedy no longer appears to work. Mr Geoffrey Bellis from Wrexham describes how his wife was advised by a friend to place a cork in her bed—with excellent results. 'After a few months a severe attack of cramp caused her to doubt the efficacy of the advice she had been given. Surprise, surprise, when she later made the bed she found the two corks on the bedroom floor.'

The practicalities of the cork treatment are described by Mrs Roger Bigley:

A few weeks ago my husband found me inserting corks under the mattress. I thought it worth a try as he had begun to leap from the bed with a cramp in the legs in the early morning. He was predictably sceptical but, I observed, did not try to stop me. How many corks and where to put them was not clear in the article I had read, so I put a few between the mattress and the frame down by his legs. There were fewer instances of cramp, but there was still the occasional

195

bout. Therefore I increased the number of corks to half a dozen, with a few a bit higher up the bed but still in the bottom half. There have been no more cramps to date.

Bedsocks: Mrs Priscilla Martin from Dublin reports: 'My husband suffers from night cramps. He was told by a physiotherapist friend to try wearing bedsocks—and it works. He wondered why he never got cramps while on holiday, but once told the cure he realized why—he wears bedsocks while on holiday because he is allergic to sheets washed in detergents!'

Avoiding milk or eating chocolate: Mr Norman Shaw, a retired surgeon, discovered by chance that his night cramps were related to his nightly consumption of milk. 'For many years I existed on a few hours' sleep at night engendered by frequent interruptions—part of the job of a consultant surgeon. On retirement I set about trying to reverse the process, not by means of pills but using tried and trusted remedies. For two years I drank half a pint of milk last thing at night. I noticed the development of very severe muscle cramps in calves and hamstrings which woke me in the small hours. Since giving up the milk there has been a complete recovery.'

On the other hand, Mr Paul Tunbridge from

Geneva reports that chocolate was curative. 'My well-qualified chemist has given me some valuable advice against the leg and foot cramps which have caused me sleepless nights. The medicine is economic and pleasant to take—black chocolate! In Switzerland this is available with 75 per cent cacao content in most stores. Two or three pieces a day keep me free from this painful condition.'

Magnets: Mrs Hilary Bonye from Kent has found that magnets have worked to prevent her cramps for over twenty years. 'I put a magnet on the affected part of my leg and the pain disappears in a few seconds. My husband, a physicist, was doubtful at first, but he agrees the effectiveness of the treatment is no coincidence.'

Further, as with Mrs Bellis's experience of corks, if the magnet is displaced, the remedy no longer works. Mrs Eileen Lynch from Suffolk uses a four-inch magnet purchased from a toyshop: 'When I had a cramp again a few nights ago, I discovered the magnet had slipped down the side of the mattress.'

Nits (Head Lice)

Head lice are remarkably resilient and persistent. No sooner have they been cleared from the hair than back they come in greater numbers than before. They are survivors and always have been. Indeed, the most ancient louse egg was discovered sticking as firmly as ever to a hair on the skull of a neolithic man who died in a cave in the Judaean desert around 6900 BC. Lice eggs, it seems, can survive anything, even the volcanic eruption of Mount Vesuvius that overwhelmed Pompeii. Chemical analysis of the remnants of the hair of a 'high-ranking young Roman woman' by an Italian archaeologist, Dr Luigi Capasso, found that even though the hard protein on the surface of the hair follicle had been destroyed by the acidity of the hot volcanic mud, the louse egg was still as firmly attached as ever.

The human head louse (*Pediculus humanus capitis*) needs the food, warmth and moisture of the scalp to survive and breed. It feeds on blood, which it obtains by piercing small blood vessels in the scalp, preventing the blood from clotting with powerful chemical secretions carried in its saliva. The claws and the light, almost transparent frame allow the head louse to move freely not just from strand to strand of hair but also—and crucially—from one head to another.

Our knowledge of the louse's behaviour has positive and negative implications for its control. The good news is that as an obligate human parasite it cannot survive for long away from the scalp and so cannot be transmitted on clothing, scarves, head gear or brushes. The bad news is that it takes only minimal contact between two heads of hair for the infestation to spread from one child to another.

The louse's resilience in the face of repeated assaults is linked to its breeding habits. The female louse produces about fifty-six eggs after just one mating; she glues these within their protective sac (the nit) to the base of a hair, almost touching the warm scalp and in which they are immune to any therapy. The lice emerge a week later, moulting their skin and reaching maturity within a fortnight. The only way of eliminating lice is to catch and eliminate the adolescents as they emerge from their nit sacs and before they are old enough to start reproducing. That is why, to be effective, any method of treatment—lotions that kill the adult louse by poisoning it, electric combs that electrocute it, and 'combing out' with hair conditioner—has to be repeated at half-weekly intervals. A systematic campaign based on any of these methods will defeat the lice. The problem is that victory can only ever be short-lived because, unless the head of every child is cleared at the same time, the infestation is likely to recur almost immediately.

The fundamental principle of home treatment, then, is the twice-weekly ritual of washing the hair, applying conditioner and 'combing out' with a nit comb to remove the adolescent lice as they emerge from their nit sacs and before they reach sexual maturity. This represents a significant improvement on earlier home remedies, as described by Mrs Elizabeth Wren from Chester during the Great War. As a young schoolgirl, she recalls, the standard treatment was 'to soak a head of long hair in paraffin and tie it up in a turban of towelling for several days. This was followed by a thorough soaking in vinegar to facilitate fine combing.'

Two other suggestions may be of help:

Lavender oil: When there is an epidemic of lice at school, it is advised that lavender oil should be applied to a child's hair line at the nape of the neck and behind the ears. This discourages the lice from jumping from one head of hair to another.

Quassia bark chips: This herbal remedy is very popular. 'Sprinkle what looks like wood chippings into a pan of water and boil until the liquid turns pale yellow. Strain and cool this astringent fluid—used as an antiseptic in the tropics—as the final rinse after washing hair. The lice loosen their grip and keel over.' Anon.

Nose Bleeds

To stop a nose bleed—as everyone knows—it is necessary to apply pressure, though the technique is important. The nose should be pinched forcefully between finger and thumb and held in that position for at least ten to fifteen minutes. For those prone to recurrent nose bleeds, the blood vessels on the inner surface of the nose need to be cauterized. While waiting for this procedure to be done, it may be sensible to purchase a swimmer's nose clip. Dr Philip Turner explains: 'This can be left in place for as long as necessary without causing too much discomfort. It does not cause the finger aching so common with manual compression. It is equally effective in children and adults and is well tolerated by the younger patient.'

There are three further 'cures' for nose bleeds:

Blood donation: The body cannot distinguish between altruistic blood loss, where the donor is giving a pint of blood, and that due to bleeding from a cut or wound. It thus responds to both by increasing the clotting mechanism of the blood. This is the probable explanation for the frequent observation that those with recurrent nose bleeds benefit from becoming blood donors, as described by Mr Paul Stickley from Hampshire. He suffered from regular and severe nose bleeds from an early age treated by regular cauterization. 'It is hard to describe the pain of having a very hot soldering iron applied to the internal lining of the nose,' he says. The turning-point came at college when Mr Stickley started to give blood 'because I thought it was a good thing to do'. Immediately he found the frequency of his nose bleeds 'reduced dramatically'.

Cold keys: Cold keys down the back of the neck is a classic old wives' tale, but the possible mechanism has been suggested by a correspondent to the *New Scientist*: 'The remedy of putting a cold bunch of keys down the patient's back may cause the blood vessels to constrict. Hence nose bleeds from rupture of tiny blood vessels in the nose can often be arrested by a sudden chill.'

A cork: It is difficult to imagine how this remedy might work (though a large cork in a small mouth may cause the nose to become 'Scrunched up', hence constricting the blood vessels within), but Mrs Sheila Springbett from Cambridgeshire reports that it is effective: 'Many years ago I attended first aid classes given by a local family doctor. He suggested the following remedy for nose bleeds. Get the patient to sit over a sink or basin and put a cork between the teeth. My son was prone to nose bleeds and it worked every time. He felt a bit silly but it was worth it. The drips soon stop.'

Palpitations

When the heart beats too fast, we experience 'palpitations'. Medical advice is necessary to identify the underlying cause, though in some cases the attack can be aborted by rubbing on the right side of the neck or by some form of shock, whether physical or electrical. Clearly there is no simple home remedy for palpitations, but the following account of one man's experience merits inclusion because it illustrates the measures some people are prepared to take to treat themselves rather than seek medical attention.

An Irish farmer was admitted to hospital after being found unconscious in his front garden. An electrocardiogram confirmed that the cause was an abnormal rhythm of the heart which rapidly resolved on conventional treatment. Once recovered, the farmer told doctors that he had suffered trauma episodes of palpitations and dizziness for almost thirty years. These, he thought, were precipitated by excitement, and he discovered that they were curable by a 'shock'. Thus, when he first got the palpitations, he would jump from a barrel and thump his feet hard on the ground when landing. This became less effective with time.

His next 'cure' was to remove his clothes, climb a ladder and jump from a considerable height into a cold-water tank on his farm. Later, he discovered that the best and simplest treatment was to grab hold of a six-volt electrified cattle-fence while simultaneously shoving the finger of his other hand into the ground to earth the shock.

The farmer was persuaded that further episodes of palpitations might be fatal, and he agreed to have a special pacemaker inserted. This recognized when his heartbeat was running at more than 155 beats a minute, at which point it administered two sharp electrical shocks to restore normal rhythm.

Piles

Piles, or haemorrhoids, are an affliction unique to humans and the roll-call of famous sufferers includes Martin Luther, Cardinal Richelieu, Copernicus and Casanova. Napoleon was a lifelong sufferer, and a particularly bad attack on the eve of Waterloo, it is alleged, was an important contributory factor to the defeat of his army by Wellington.

Piles are caused by the prolapse of the veins around the anal canal which are then pinched tight by the muscles of the anal sphincter, resulting in bleeding and intense pain. A standard treatment available from the chemist without prescription is a cream containing a mild steroid and a local anaesthetic such as Anugesic. There are in addition a range of home remedies that can be tried.

Ice: Cold constricts the blood vessels as well as having a local anaesthetic effect. The person with piles is advised to sit naked on a chair on which has been placed ice cubes (or a packet of frozen vegetables) wrapped in a clean towel or two, as advised by John Rudkin of Cambridgeshire: 'Two towels should be used to insulate the piles from the bag of frozen vegetables which should be at around 20°F. After wrenching my knee playing squash I gave it the frozen vegetable treatment (using one towel) and ended up with mild frostbite. Piles would be more sensitive to such an insult!'

Miss E.J.N. Willis from Suffolk has devised a much more user-friendly way of applying the ice treatment to the delicate area: 'Buy a pack of the small dry discs sold for the removal of facial make-up. Thoroughly moisten the individual pads with water, spread out on a plastic tray and place in the freezer or ice-making compartment of the fridge. When frozen use daily after the usual evacuation routine, applying for about two minutes until melting begins. Repeat at bedtime if helpful.'

Laxatives: Constipation can, by causing straining at stool, precipitate an attack of piles, while the pain of piles, by discouraging defecation, can cause constipation. In either situation, loosening the stool and increasing its bulk with a high fluid intake and fibre is an appropriate treatment (see Constipation, page 91).

Vaseline: A thin layer of Vaseline or petroleum jelly just inside the anus will ease the passage of the stool and thus relieve pain on defecation.

Mistletoe: Mr J.R. from Hertfordshire reports: 'After a hectic time preparing for Christmas, my dreaded haemorrhoids returned. I recently read that mistletoe was a suggested cure, so I thought why not. My local friendly florist was pleased to give me the berries waiting to be thrown away. After washing them and applying between two pieces of gauze, I experienced wonderful relief and a complete cure. The moral is—have your haemorrhoids over Christmas.'

Restless Legs

Restless legs syndrome is an obscure affliction in which an unpleasant creeping sensation is felt deep within the bone and muscle. 'It feels as if my whole leg is full of small worms,' is how one sufferer describes it, and to another it is 'as if ants are running up and down my bones'. Movement of the legs provides the only solace, and sufferers find it impossible to keep still. This torture is psychological as well as physical. The creeping may persist for hours at a time, keeping the tormented victim up till four or five in the morning, and this forced insomnia unsettles the mind, inducing hallucinations and depression.

Medical examination of sufferers reveals no abnormality; nor do other investigatory tests. No abnormalities of muscles or nerves have ever been identified. The cause is unknown, though it is presumed that there must be some area deep in the brain from which the crawling sensation originates.

Those who suffer from restless legs will get little help from their doctors who are as mystified by the complaint as their patients, and for which until recently they had no certain cure to offer. Ropinirole, a drug originally developed for the treatment of Parkinson's disease, when given at a small dose of 0.5 mg three times a day, has been reported by many sufferers to be highly efficacious. Several contributors have, however, suggested a variety of home remedies which could be tried.

Heat: Heat in the form of a hot bath last thing

at night or a hot-water bottle and bedsocks can prevent restless legs. Blessed relief is sometimes reported during a viral illness such as flu which, by raising the temperature, provides solace for a few days.

Cold: Alternatively, some sufferers find relief by pouring icy water over their legs, lying horizontal on the ground and sticking their feet in the refrigerator, or, weather permitting, walking barefoot in the snow. Less drastically, a doctor from North London writes: 'I remove all the bedding from my legs and allow them to cool. After about thirty minutes the sensation of restless legs subsides and I can cover up and go to sleep.'

Exercise: 'Lie on the floor and "cycle" in the air until the muscles ease up.' Anon.

Cramp: Fascinatingly, deliberately inducing an attack of cramp can bring relief, as described by Mr J.I. Visser from Edinburgh: 'Having been driven up the wall (literally) with restless legs and tried everything, eventually out of desperation I pulled my calf muscles so tight that very quickly I got cramp in the leg. Letting go, I immediately noticed the infernal irritation had just about disappeared. Now when I feel the restless legs are about to start up again, I induce a cramp, let go immediately and have no more trouble. Sometimes I have

208

to repeat the process a few times but no more.'

Water: Emeritus surgeon Mr T. P.N. Jenkins from Surrey reports that he has been 'plagued by restless legs from my late teens into my eighties. It was a great event in my life when I discovered a simple solution—a drink of water. As the discomfort of restless legs impinges on sleep, a point is reached when it is well worthwhile to get out of bed and drink. In a few minutes, the symptoms ease off and a deep sleep returns.'

Rosacea

Rosacea, or acne rosacea, is best conceived of as a form of acne whose symptoms can none the less be devastating. In the words of one 36-year-old sufferer: 'The problem is that I have an extremely hot and red face and very bloodshot eyes. It is a total catastrophe. I am unable to work, I have no social life or friends, cannot travel and find it difficult to do anything that most people would take as normal. I can be outdoors in a cool breeze and I can just about cope, but any time there is the slightest rise in temperature, such as indoors, I just get hotter and ever more red.'

As with so many conditions, the cause of rosacea is not precisely known and there seems to be no surefire cure, despite the offer almost one hundred years ago of a $100,000 reward by the American financier J. Pierpoint Morgan, who himself suffered from rosacea. Its early symptoms include a ready predisposition to blushing, especially following alcohol. Subsequently the face is permanently reddened with small acne-type pustules.

The standard medical treatment, which works for many, is the antibiotic tetracycline taken by mouth or applied directly to the face. This usually has to be taken for long periods. A reader from Layburn writes:

My husband has suffered from rosacea for many years. He has always had a 'good' colour, but it became more and more noticeable in his late thirties and early forties. His face will get redder and redder after drinking alcohol, being in a warm room, etc. He was a flautist in a Guards band. One day he bumped into his medical officer, his face was feeling especially hot and he was immediately sent to the military hospital at Millbank. The specialist told him what the trouble was, put him on tetracycline and impressed on him that he must always repeat this course every six months. This he has done for over thirty years and it has never failed to take effect.

Some cases of rosacea, it is now believed,

may be due to a sensitivity to a bacterium found in the gut, *Helicobacter*, which causes gastritis and ulcers. Certainly, eradicating *Helicobacter* with antibiotics has in some cases been followed by a marked improvement. Further suggestions include:

Simple washing: Many of those who have rosacea are keen to emphasize the need to avoid potential precipitating factors in soaps and creams that are applied to the face. One reader found water to be actively therapeutic: 'I have found that frequent bathing of the face and eyes with cool water always helps.'

Cotton pillow: Switching to a cotton pillow can result in a marked improvement of the symptoms, but it is noted that 'its case should be washed only in very hot water, not with soap or detergent'.

Diet: It is only sensible to cut out flush-inducing foods and drinks such as alcohol and spicy curries. It is reported that giving up coffee can produce a marked improvement in symptoms.

Ultraviolet light: Dr Alan Ure, an analytical chemist from the University of Strathclyde, writes:

As a semi-retired scientist of seventy-two,

211

I have begun to suffer from not too severe attacks of acne rosacea with reddening of the skin over the cheekbones, bridge and tip of the nose and forehead. This was often accompanied by micro-pimples. I assumed, having noted that those parts of the forehead covered by a flap of hair seemed unaffected, that ultraviolet light was at least a contributory factor (but certainly not the only one). Treatment with a thin daily application of ultraviolet protective cream (factor 15) to the affected areas completely suppressed the condition. Stopping the application brings about a recurrence of the problem.

Facial massage: The 'boggy' nature of the skin in rosacea is due to the accumulation of fluid. A Danish dermatologist, Paul Sobye, claimed back in 1950 that this could be dispersed by regular facial massage: 'We rejoice in favourable results,' he wrote rather quaintly. The benefits, however, may not become apparent until after three months of treatment.

Sex Selection

Many couples nowadays having had two children of the same sex are keen to have another—but only if it is of the opposite sex.

There is thus a natural interest in the question of whether in some way or another couples might be able to influence the sex of their offspring by sex selection. This can be readily achieved by antenatal diagnosis, which by determining the sex of the foetus makes it possible to abort any of the 'wrong' sex. Such a practice is luckily outlawed in Britain, so couples must resort to other means for which, though they certainly sound ingenious, there is no serious evidence of their effectiveness.

The sex of a child is determined by whether the ovum is fertilized by a sperm whose twenty-three chromosomes include either the female sex X chromosome or the male sex Y chromosome. They are called X and Y because of their shape, and the only physical difference between the two is that the Y chromosome is missing one arm's length so the sperm carrying it is infinitesimally slightly less heavy. Clearly, if sex selection is to work, it is necessary to separate the two types of sperm, and there must be some other distinguishing physical characteristic that allows this to be done.

In 1979 Dr Landrum Shettles, an American gynaecologist, reported that Y-bearing sperm swim faster and so, other things being equal, they should get to the ovum first and many more boys than girls would be conceived. But this is balanced, he claimed, by the fact that the X-bearing female sperm, though less speedy, are more resilient and so less likely to be destroyed by vaginal secretions which are more acidic around the crucial time of ovulation.

If this theory is correct, then it is possible to practice do-it-yourself sex selection.

For a girl: Couples wishing to have a girl should first douche the vagina with a diluted teaspoonful of acidic white vinegar which will selectively 'knock off' the competing sperm carrying the male Y chromosome. In addition they should be sure to have sexual intercourse immediately around the time of ovulation, which can be determined by a slight rise in body temperature and the presence of a clear, jelly-like vaginal discharge. This gives the sperm carrying the female X chromosome an equal chance against the male.

For a boy: By contrast, couples who wish to have a boy should douche the vagina with a diluted alkaline solution of sodium bicarbonate, thus rendering the environment less hostile to the male X-bearing sperm. In addition sexual activity should occur either just before or just after ovulation to maximize on the Y-bearing sperm's ability to swim faster.

Dr Shettles subsequently proposed a further modification based on the observation that when the woman has an orgasm her vaginal secretions tend to be alkaline, and so only those wishing to have a boy should try to achieve this pleasurable plateau.

Dr Shettles has sold a lot of books describing his techniques, presumably because even if the method is completely valueless, half of all the couples following his advice would by chance end up with a child of their desired sex.

Shingles

Shingles, which is caused by the same virus as chicken pox, is known by the Norwegians as 'the belt of roses from hell' and by the Danes more simply as 'hell fire'. Both names evoke its most salient feature—shingles can be very painful indeed. The rash disappears after a week or so but the stabbing, toothache-like pain in the sensory nerve endings can persist for months. This may require very powerful analgesics up to and including morphine.

Further, the site of the rash can become incredibly sensitive, for which a reader from Hove devised the following home remedy. 'The pain can be quite agonizing during the day as one's clothing "dances" on the skin at every slight movement. Painkillers have little effect. In desperation to keep clothing away from my skin, I tried a large plastic bag attached to my back with five pieces of

Sellotape! This, of course, provided a defence against clothing and seemed like a miracle cure—and only necessary during the day. It has a slightly "crinkly" sound as one moves around, but is barely noticeable. We visited Windsor Castle while I was wearing my "cure" and got no strange looks!'

Sinusitis (Catarrh)

The sinuses are large, air-filled holes in the skull on either side of the nose. Their prime function is to humidify and warm air on its way down to the lungs, half filtering out bacteria and other particular matter. They themselves are thus vulnerable to infection from these bacteria, becoming filled with a sort of infected glue that drips down the back of the nose, causing sufferers to wake in the morning with a vile taste in the mouth. The head feels heavy, headaches are common and there is a curious deadening of the mental function, making it difficult to concentrate.

This glue, better known as catarrh, blocks both the nasal passages and the opening into the sinuses at the back of the nose, thus preventing the circulation of air through them. Self-evidently, then, unblocking the nose by dislodging the catarrh should be beneficial.

Steam inhalation: Steam inhalation is the

cheapest and most effective of remedies and should be used much more frequently. It is certainly preferable to the decongestant medications procured at considerable cost from the local chemist. Boiling water is placed in a shallow pan to which a drop of menthol or eucalyptus oil may be added and a towel is placed over the head. After fifteen minutes of steam inhalation, the nostrils will be clear—at least for a while. Some people prefer to go to the bathroom, close the windows, place a towel against the door and sit on the side of the bath inhaling the steam from a really hot bath or shower.

Salt: Mr Alan Woodcock from Grimsby reports:

I had just started my final year for the London matriculation exam when I became listless, started experiencing severe headaches and my nose seemed to be permanently blocked. My local doctor sent me to see an ENT specialist who, after X-rays, decided that I needed a sinus operation as my nasal passages were blocked. I returned home to await hospital admission.

The next day our local vet arrived to give our dog its half-yearly dose of 'jollop' (his phrase). Seeing my predicament, he said, "What you need, my boy, is to cover a sixpence with salt and dry bicarbonate of soda. Tip each into a saucer and dissolve them in boiled water. As soon as it is cool enough, stick your nose in the liquid and sniff."

It wasn't a pleasant experience, but after several minutes of sniffing, first one giant sneeze then another brought out large hard cores of 'nasal mucus'. A painful experience, but the relief was worth it.

Two or three weeks later, I attended the hospital for admission. After telling the specialist of my cure, I was sent for further X-rays and told I could go home. My nasal passages were now completely clear.

A variant of this remedy is reported by Mr Barclay Hankin from Sussex: 'Take a small quantity of ordinary table salt and place dry on palm of hand. Take a similar quantity of dry sodium bicarbonate (baking powder); place next to the salt and mix. Sniff up the most blocked nostril! This will sting rather unpleasantly but will help to unblock it. Repeat with other nostril or until cured. Once or twice should do the trick.'

A swim: This is a variant of the salt remedy, and is described by Mrs J.F. Edwards from Huntingdon: 'One very hot summer day at the

218

seaside all my family decided to go for a swim—but I had a very bad attack of sinusitis. They got ready to go in, so I decided I would go too, never mind tomorrow! Tomorrow came and my sinusitis was no more. So needless to say, after that when I had an attack, I would go for a swim.

Food sensitivity: There is no doubt that certain foods can predispose to formation of catarrh; the main culprit is undoubtedly dairy products. A reader reports how her daughter inadvertently discovered that milk was a causative factor:

My daughter suffered from sinus problems badly in her teens and early twenties, needing or rather being prescribed a variety of drugs that did little for her and some which made her worse. When she decided to leave home and have a flat of her own she was very short of cash. In an effort to cut every bill she could she opted to have skimmed milk instead of whole milk, which was dearer. She got through the winter with no sinusitis or any related problems. Better finances meant she went back to whole milk and back came the sinus problems. Back on skimmed milk, and the problem disappeared. So a change of milk meant lower milk bills, no prescription charges, no wasting doctors' time, and no sick leave for her. Perhaps it will work for others.

Humans, it would seem, are not the only ones who are sensitive to dairy products in this way, as Dr Layinka Swinburne reports in the *Lancet*:

The patient, aged fifteen, has had a cough for at least five years and a constantly running nose with a discharge of thick mucus. Her voice became hoarse and very often she could only mouth her messages silently. Many therapies were tried including antibiotics, both in short courses and longer low-dose regimens. Over the past year no treatment has had much effect. I realized that if she had two legs instead of four I would be considering a diagnosis of milk allergy. We stopped her daily treat of a saucer of cream at coffee time which she had learned to demand in a special voice. In forty-eight hours her nose dried up, the cough stopped completely, she could purr without bringing on a bout of coughing.'

A further if more unlikely culprit is orange juice, as described by Mr J.B. Roberts from Nottingham:

Some time ago I used to suffer from very severe nasal congestion. I tried all sorts of tablets but they only gave temporary relief. Then by chance I had to go away on a course for about a week, and to and behold the congestion cleared up. I sat down and had a think about what I had eaten or drunk at this hotel and how it differed from what I normally have at home. By a process of elimination it turned out, to my utter astonishment, to be orange juice. Even an eggcupful would set it off. It came as a bit of a blow as I was very fond of this drink. The cure was instantaneous.

Skin Ulcers

Poor circulation or varicose veins predisposes to ulcers of the skin especially in the older age group. The standard treatment includes dressing the ulcers and elevating the affected parts, but they can be very slow to heal. The value of honey in these circumstances was first recorded by the Egyptians in 2000 BC (see 'The Evidence', page 13), and as Mr P. J. Armon, a consultant gynaecologist, reports, the use of honey continues to this day:

Honey has been used in the treatment of infected wounds at the Kilimanjaro

Medical Centre in Tanzania for the past four years with excellent results. In one case a woman was admitted with a massive post-partum haemorrhage, requiring an emergency hysterectomy and five further operations to deal with intestinal obstruction and abscesses. During the course of this debilitating illness she developed a massive bedsore on her sacrum, 15–20 centimetres in size, exposing the bone. The surface of the sore was covered, three times daily, with a thin layer of pure honey and a dry dressing. Twenty-one days later, the cavity had closed without surgical treatment and the sacrum was covered in a new layer of skin. Only one seven-day course of antibiotics had been used during this time.

Honey was also an important aspect of the treatment devised by the famous plastic surgeon, Sir Archibald MacIndoe, for treating the burn injuries sustained by pilots during the Battle of Britain. Mrs K. Henderson from Evesham recalls:

Ever since I visited the late Dr MacIndoe's hospital in East Grinstead to see a Spitfire pilot badly burned in the Battle of Britain—he was shrouded in thick bandages and honey—I have used pure honey on wounds. Recently I developed a leg ulcer and was treated for two months by the district nurse using wet dressings and Vaseline bandages. It didn't get better at all, so I put on a dry gauze with honey. Twenty-four hours later it was half the size and after three days—and more honey—it had completely gone! Much to the fury of the district nurse!

Mrs Elaine Field from Cornwall records a similar if less dramatic result. 'I have had for six months or more flaky skin on the top joint of my ring finger. After being given some hydrocortisone ointment by the chemist, I then had a huge weeping sore which my doctor thought might be cancerous and accordingly referred me to a specialist. In the meantime, my finger looked so awful that I had to cover the sore when I left the house, and each time I smeared honey over the patch. Within two weeks it was completely clear and has not returned. I consider honey to be a miracle cure.'

Smelly Scalp Syndrome

This mysterious symptom was originally described by a 43-year-old reader: 'Since my first baby seventeen years ago, I have suffered from a smelly scalp,' she writes. 'I wash my hair every day, sometimes twice, but after only a few hours my scalp feels as though it has not been washed for days and has an embarrassingly greasy smell. I have had two more children and the problem has persisted, getting worse when my period is due.' Her own doctor she describes as being 'totally uninterested'.

Several home remedies for this unusual problem have been suggested:

Wash less: A reader from Liverpool implicates antidandruff shampoos, since the scalp reacts to regular hairwashing by secreting ever-greater quantities of greasy sebum: 'Normally my hair needs only a weekly wash,' she writes. When she started using a strong shampoo, 'my hair became lank and greasy after a day. It took six months to get back to normal.'

Food sensitivity: Mrs Madeline Phillips from Kent reports: 'Several years ago, my husband noticed that my scalp had an unpleasant odour even though I was washing my hair daily.' Her physiotherapist (Mrs Phillips also has painful joints) suggested that she might be allergic to dairy products. So, 'I now drink goat's milk and try not to eat so much butter and cheese.' Her husband no longer complains about her hair odour and, as a bonus, her joint pains and stiffness 'have also greatly improved'.

Hormonal: There might well be a hormonal component to the complaint, because greasy hair, together with acne, can be a sign of overproduction of the sex hormone testosterone. One woman who had 'suffered from smelly scalp for most of my life', reported that 'it disappeared as soon as I started taking HRT. I no longer have to wash my hair daily (and it looks and smells better). It's wonderful.'

Sneezing

Sneezing is particularly useful for dislodging irritating particles from the nose. It has two distinct phases. In the first, the lining of the nose responds to some irritating particle by becoming engorged and secreting a clear mucous substance in which the particle will be expelled. The nasal engorgement in turn stimulates a series of rapid, deep breaths drawing a large volume of air within the chest. The second phase starts once the pressure of the lungs has passed the critical point, when the combination of the elastic recoil of lung tissue and the contraction of muscle in the chest and abdominal wall hurtles air back out of the lungs at a speed of a hundred feet per second, expelling the mucus droplets containing the irritating particles in a fine mist to a distance of around six feet.

Rhinitis, or chronic inflammation of the lining of the nose, will then, naturally enough, result in repetitive sneezing. Much the commonest cause is allergy to pollen resulting in hay fever, or when the rhinitis is not just confined to the summer months but throughout the year, some other allergen. Medical treatment is straightforward and involves regular use of a steroid nasal spray. Prevention with honey desensitization and decongestion with steam inhalation is described in the section on hay fever (see page 138).

There is another type of repetitive sneezing, however, usually in association with coughing, described by Mr G. Haddon from Kent as 'an itching, tickling in the throat which brings on convulsive coughing, often ending in about six almighty sneezes. This is accompanied by aching ears, a feeling in the nose and head as of a nasty cold but no or little production of mucus. A bout can last about one or two minutes and can come on at any time but particularly during the evening and at night.'

Repetitive sneezing is usually induced by

one or other of the following precipitants:

Alcohol: Mrs Beatrice Urquhart from Surrey reports:

> My husband used to make wine from an assortment of packs. Latterly he has been buying cases of different supermarket 'plonk'. He reckons the plonk on special offer is nearly as cheap as making wine and without all the hassle. Gradually I have come to realize that my spasmodic, compulsive projectile sneezing used to be caused by a particular batch of my husband's home brew and it is now caused by some (but not by all) types of the wine he buys. When we entertain, we serve good-quality wine, so it is very rarely that I have to embarrass our guests by having one of my horrific, explosive sneezing attacks.

Aspirin: Professor Sir Donald Harrison, past President of the Royal Society of Medicine, reports that his wife developed repetitive sneezing. When a small amount of ground-up aspirin was placed up her nose at an allergy clinic, it promptly precipitated an attack.

Chocolate: Mr Donald Bell from Norwich reports that his first job on leaving school was as a taster in a chocolate factory: 'Gradually I began to experience attacks of sneezing. They became more violent as time passed. I could saturate a handkerchief in a matter of minutes.' He chanced upon an article in which an American dentist claimed that sugar was associated with repetitive sneezing: 'From that time I refused, so far as my duties allowed, consumption of confectionary and gave up voluntarily sugar in tea and coffee. To my great relief my symptoms quickly disappeared.'

Newsprint: Mrs Dorothy Castle from Birmingham reports the experience of her friend 'who has similar symptoms every evening when she opens her evening paper'.

In each case, treatment requires avoiding the precipitating factor, and if this is not possible, a steroid nasal spray may be needed. In addition, Mrs H. Wale from Warwickshire recommends salt: 'Just put a few grains of salt in the palm of your hand, then lick off and swallow. This provides immediate relief and has been a great blessing.'

Snoring

The nearest most people come to murdering their partners or spouses is when they are woken yet again by stentorian snoring from the adjoining pillow. Snoring is no laughing matter; it can wreck relationships, disrupt families and indeed be harmful to health. A heavy snorer suffers from chronic exhaustion and is more prone to heart ailments.

Snoring occurs when the tissues at the back of the throat, in sleep, collapse inwards, so that air has to pass through a very narrow aperture—producing the characteristic grunting sounds. In its most severe form, the narrowing at the back of the throat can be so complete that breathing may stop altogether—a condition known as obstructive sleep apnoea or OSA. A person with OSA is, as it were, suffering from self-strangulation—the oxygen concentration in the blood falls to a point where the breathing centre in the brain is stimulated to make another voluntary intake of breath.

Those with OSA get insufficient restful sleep—they wake with a headache in the morning, are sleepy during the day and fall asleep at the slightest opportunity, whether at work, in church or while driving a car and sometimes in the middle of a meal.

Heavy snoring is a potentially serious condition that needs proper medical evaluation. There are several simple remedies, however, each working in a different way, that can alleviate or abolish snoring, thus obviating the need for more drastic measures.

Cut down on alcohol: There is no harm in a couple of glasses of wine in the evening and even a nightcap, but serious drinking in the evening is a major contributory factor to snoring for two reasons: a lot of alcohol in the bloodstream at night reduces the body's movements when asleep while simultaneously suppressing the breathing centre in the brain. Thus the typical position of the hard-drinking heavy snorer is of a person flat on his back emitting deep intermittent grunts.

Lose weight: This is, of course, easier said than done, but reducing the amount of body fat all over will also reduce the thickness of the tissues at the back of the throat and thus there is less to collapse inwards to obstruct the inflow of breath.

Steam: Nasal stuffiness is a potent cause of snoring by preventing breathing through the nose, so all the air that is inhaled and exhaled has to go through the mouth. Hence those with a cold or hay fever tend to be heavy snorers, and it is only sensible to clear and open up the nasal passages at night by placing hot water in a flat pan, throwing a towel over the head and breathing in and out for ten minutes.

Marbles: Dr George McGeary from Oregon describes this interesting snoring cure. 'It was suggested by my mother who sewed a small glass marble into the pyjama top between the shoulder blades under a scrap of cloth. When the snorer rolls on his back, he immediately rolls back on his side usually without waking and resumes sleep without snoring. Once a marble is sewn into the pyjamas it can be forgotten about—as they go through the wash without problems.'

Dr Fritz Shmerl, a physician from California, has suggested a variant on this theme: 'I advise the use of half a soft sponge rubber ball six centimetres in diameter. Such a ball is available in any toyshop. Its hemisphere is detached and fastened to the mid part of the back of the pyjama tops. I use friction material such as Velcro that when glued to the flat disc of the half-ball clings firmly to the pyjamas fitted with a complementary piece.'

Cotton wool: The alternative to treating the snorer is to treat the partner. When the ears are plugged with cotton wool at night, the sounds of snoring become much fainter and sleep is no longer disturbed.

Sore Throat

Family doctors will, on average, see four patients with a sore throat each week. This adds up to around 150,000 consultations a year in Britain, for which doctors prescribe £22.5 million worth of antibiotics. This may be appropriate where there is obviously a bacterial infection, usually caused by the bug Streptococcus. Here the back of the throat is grossly inflamed with signs of pus or an abscess, the throat glands are enlarged and painful and the temperature is raised.

In most cases, however, the cause of the sore throat is a virus which does not respond to antibiotics and so will simply get better of its own accord. Here the best treatment is to control the main symptoms of pain and swelling; and simple remedies, by avoiding the hazards of inappropriate antibiotics, are clearly useful. The efficacy of the 'cold cloth' cure—advocated by several contributors—is of particular interest as most people (and doctors) are unaware of it.

Salt and water gargle: Gargling with salt and water, or with an antiseptic such as TCP, three or four times a day will sterilize the back of the throat and promote healing of the inflamed tissues. It is perhaps less well appreciated that both soluble aspirin and spirits such as whisky or brandy have a local anaesthetic effect, so regular gargling with these remedies will reduce the pain associated with a sore throat.

Lemon juice and honey: This combination is an excellent remedy for sore throats; the astringent, antiseptic properties of the lemon are offset by the soothing (and anti-infective) effects of the honey. They should be mixed together in hot water or tea and sipped throughout the day.

Egg and sugar: Mrs Patricia Snell from Somerset reports: 'I often use this sore throat remedy with my family: stiffly beat an egg white to which you add sugar (and for small children, a little pink colouring). This meringue mixture can be eaten by the spoonful and is most soothing. I suppose there must be a healing property in the albumen of the egg.'

Hot milk and suet: Mrs Jane Garrard from Dorset recommends grating raw suet onto a cup of hot milk for a sore throat. 'The suet coats the throat and helps it to heal. During the war, my two-year-old son had a heavy cold and when he woke crying in the evening I would give him the hot milk and suet and he would return to bed and sleep till morning.'

Cold cloth cure: One reader's father was a chemist. The family lived on the shop premises so there was plenty of medical treatment to hand, but none the less her mother's favourite remedy was the cold towel treatment: 'A large handkerchief was wrung out in cold water, laid around the neck and covered with a woollen scarf on retiring to bed. So far as I can remember, it always worked.' Mrs Margaret Bellord from Hertfordshire also testifies to this treatment, pointing out in particular that the water has to be very cold. As the cloth warmed up, 'It was horribly uncomfortable . . . but it worked.'

It is not clear whether the cold water aspect of this treatment is strictly necessary, however, for as Mrs Janet Allen of West Sussex points out: 'At grammar school in the 1950s we wore long woollen knee socks. If we had a sore throat, the remedy was to wrap a worn (i.e., unwashed) sock around the neck overnight. In the morning the sore throat had gone!'

Vaseline: Vaseline or petroleum jelly has a soothing effect on sore throats, as Mr G.W.J. Crawford's uncle discovered while serving in Burma during the last war:

> He developed a severe sore throat such that he was quite unable to swallow. It appeared that he would choke to death, as he was having difficulty in breathing too. His first aid kit contained the ubiquitous field dressing—no help there— and a jar of Vaseline, slightly runny in the intense heat. In desperation, he put a teaspoonful of Vaseline into his mouth. Amazingly it went down, giving some instant relief, and the soreness and swelling began to disappear quite quickly.

By the next day, after another dose, the throat was much better—and soon all was quite well.

Allergy: One of the symptoms of hay fever can be a sore throat, and for those in whom the condition is chronic or persistent the possibility of some allergen should be considered, as Mr Fred Small of Lancashire reports:

I used to go to work, sit in my office and by about ten o'clock each day I used to start getting a slight sore throat and my voice was affected. This grew worse as the day went on. In the evening at home, the problem would subside and by morning I was normal again. This went on for a year or more. I saw an ENT specialist who could find nothing wrong. Then my secretary saw a television programme about ferns that give off spores which are invisible to the naked eye and which float about in the room. These can affect some people. I had a large fern in my office. The fern was removed and I was cured immediately!

Splinters

The conventional method of removing splinters —with a sterilized safety pin—causes some discomfort which can be avoided with the following remedy, suggested by Jane Morgan from Leigh on Sea. 'The solution to the removal of a splinter has been used in my family for many years successfully. You simply put some soft soap (from underneath the tablet which somebody always leaves floating in the bath) on a piece of lint. Add a small amount of brown sugar (it must be brown), place over the site of the splinter and stick down firmly. Leave overnight and, hey presto, the splinter will be on the lint in the morning.

Independent confirmation of this striking remedy comes from Mrs Mary Rosewarne from Howe who tried it out on a splinter she had had in her finger for five days. 'The following morning, as I removed the plaster from my finger, the splinter actually started "rising" like a worm coming straight up out of the ground.' Mr K. Bale from Lincoln comments that the 'soft' soap and 'brown' sugar are not necessary: 'Ordinary soap and sugar are equally effective.'

Split Skin

Splitting of the skin causes painful fissures (colloquially known as hacks), most often at the tips of the fingers or around the heel. There are several good proprietary preparations including 'New Skin' which one contributor says should be 'painted over a whisp of cotton wool placed over the crack first'. Two other popular remedies are as follows:

Superglue: Mr J.C. Clarke, a retired anaesthetist from Belfast, reports that 'painful fissures can be instantly rendered painless by the use of superglue. The fissures should be clean and dry. Carefully fill the open fissure with bubble-free superglue and allow to dry. As healing takes place, the scab falls away spontaneously.' However, Mrs Mary Elliott from Essex was not so impressed. 'The superglue certainly healed the crack, but a few days later the skin around the thumb started to peel away all the way down to the first joint.'

Sellotape: Mr David Fairburn from Argyle reports: 'I have suffered for many of my sixty-eight years from "hacks". Some years ago in frustration I wound myself up in Sellotape—the hacks were completely cured in a matter of hours. Being quite unscientific, I proceeded to treat some of the hacks with the tape and to leave others untreated. The untreated hacks remained for days but the treated ones cured without exception overnight.'

Vitamin E: This is not strictly a home remedy, but several readers have commented on its efficacy: 'For about three or four years I have

237

suffered each winter from deep bleeding cracks on my fingertips and on the soles of my feet. I have now been taking vitamin supplements for about three weeks—60 mg per day—and they have all healed up. I am so grateful!' Mrs Margaret Reynolds from Croydon.

Sprains

The common form of ankle sprain is known as an 'inversion injury', when the foot inverts inwards and with the full weight of the body now being taken by the ligaments on the outer side of the ankle, they tear. Swelling and bruising follow soon afterwards. Prompt application of ice over the injured ligaments provides both relief from the pain and reduces the degree of swelling, but these injuries can take up to six weeks to heal.

There is a further type of ankle injury due to the misplacement of the small bones of the foot that is often mistaken for an inversion injury but which can be promptly relieved by manipulation or a sudden jolting movement. This is described by Mr Richard Bailey from Kent who, while bowling in a cricket match, ran into a depression in the pitch and 'badly turned' his ankle. He had to be carried off the pitch and continued to hobble about until on a short walk the following evening, 'I spied some ripe fruit in an orchard and climbed over a six-foot-high gate intending to scrump some. I fell heavily down on the other side, feet first, and immediately the ankle was painless and fully operational again. What a joy that moment was!'

Mrs Marie Cottrell from Edinburgh tells a similar story. 'I sprained my ankle and foot very badly, attended hospital and was told to treat it gently. I did so for weeks but it was still painful when I walked, however gingerly. Then one day when crossing the road, a car came racing round the bend towards me and I had to run for my life. When I put my foot down hard to run, I felt it ripple and it was as if a piece of jigsaw had been put back into place. My foot felt much better and was soon back to normal.'

Dr J. Nickson, a retired family doctor and skilled manipulator from Berkshire, explains: 'The small joints in the forefoot become locked in malposition when the foot is twisted. If this is the case, manipulation of the forefoot produces a good "click" or "pop" and the condition is immediately relieved.'

Stings

BEES, WASPS AND HORNETS

Bees, wasps and hornets inject their venom under the skin causing redness, swelling and pain which can last several hours unless prompt action is taken. The standard advice for bee stings has been that the barb should be flicked off with a knife or other sharp object, but this, it now appears, is not the case, for reasons outlined by Dr Kirk Visscher of the University of California. 'The advice that people should be concerned about how bee stings are removed is counter-productive. The precise method of removal is irrelevant, as even slight delays in removal caused by concern over the correct procedure, or finding an appropriate implement, are likely to increase the dose of venom received. The advice should simply be to emphasize that a bee sting should be removed as quickly as possible.'

Honey-bee stings are of particular concern because they can attract other bees to sting the victim. Dr Visscher comments: 'The most important response to bees defending their nests should be to get away from the vicinity as quickly as possible. An alarm chemical is emitted at the base of the honey-bee sting; when detected by other bees, it leads them in

240

localizing the victim and makes them more likely to sting. In such a situation, reaching safety is much more important than removing the sting immediately.'

By contrast, it is recommended that the immediate response to a wasp sting should be to suck it out before the hole closes up. 'Father always said he could taste the bitterness if it was done in time. You should, of course, spit it out,' writes Mrs Marian Banyard from Suffolk. It is also claimed that as wasp venom is slightly alkaline and bee venom is acidic, so the specific antidotes will be different. Wasp stings may be neutralized by acid-containing substances such as onion and vinegar, while bee stings are helped by alkaline compounds such as sodium bicarbonate (baking powder).

There are thus a variety of home remedies to choose from.

Cold: Ice cubes placed on the sting have a local anaesthetic effect, reduce the swelling and prevent the spread of the venom. Stings in the mouth or throat can be alleviated by sucking on an ice cube. If there is the slightest sign of difficulty in breathing then prompt medical attention should be sought.

Heat: Heat in the form of a hot flannel or hairdryer directed at the sting may be equally effective as cold, as indeed may be cigarettes. In the words of Mr Eric Wardrope from the

Dordogne area of France, whose wife is allergic to wasp stings: 'The local people of this area always keep cigarettes and matches handy. When stung, light a cigarette and hold it as close to the sting as comfort allows. Keep it there until it has burnt the whole length. This stops the poison spreading and saves a lot of discomfort. We are non-smokers but always keep cigarettes in the medicine cabinet, the car and my wife's handbag for such an emergency.'

Onion: The value of onions in treating wasp stings has been recognized since 1775 when the following note was published in the *Norwich Mercury*: 'As wasps are this summer very numerous, it may be of some Utility to the Public to be informed that Onion juice, gently swallowed, is a certain Remedy for the Sting of Wasp in the Throat, an Accident that has been often known to prove fatal.'

The supposed beneficial effect of countering the alkalinity of a wasp sting with acidic compounds is outlined above. Whatever the precise explanation, many attest to its efficacy: 'Many years ago, when my children were small, we were on holiday in Wales when my wife was stung on the arm by a wasp. We called in at a nearby cottage and begged an onion which rapidly dealt with it. Subsequently, while my children were growing up, I always carried an onion and a knife in the car during the summer season.' Mr Stanley Green from Cambridge.

'In the 1930s I used to help at Girl Guide camp. Outside the cookhouse there was always a string of onions hanging in case anyone was stung by a wasp, especially on the lips or top of the throat. If this happened to a girl, she had to bite an onion to relieve the pain.' Mrs Agnes Bantock from Hertfordshire.

Vinegar: Mrs Grant Norton from Buckinghamshire points out that 'vinegar dabbed onto the sting with a small wad of cotton wool is much simpler than the onion therapy. It can also be swallowed as a small teaspoonful or on a sugar lump.'

Toothpaste: Mrs B. Lutyens from Doverton writes: 'For years I have used toothpaste on wasp stings. It is usually on hand and is instantly effective. I am not a crank. I live in the depths of the country, and so long as I take toothpaste on a picnic it is a useful solution to these unpleasant stings.'

Mud: For those in the countryside without access to hot water or ice cubes, a paste of earth and water covered with a bandage is recommended.

Sodium bicarbonate (baking powder): A paste of water and sodium bicarbonate has a favourable soothing effect on bee stings by countering their acidity.

SCORPION STINGS

Mrs T.M. Godber from Somerset reports the following remedy for scorpion stings from the time she lived in a rubber planter's bungalow in Malaya. 'My younger sister stood on a scorpion and was stung on the sole of the foot. It was New Year's Eve and we all thought she would be unable to enjoy the dance that evening to celebrate the occasion. Our Chinese cook volunteered a proven antidote. We crushed the scorpion and applied it to the wound, bandaging it in place. She had scarcely any swelling or discomfort and was able to enjoy the dance as planned.'

Equally unusual, Mr H.M. Burkill from Surrey recalls the following remedy for scorpion stings from his time as a prisoner of war of the Japanese on the infamous Burma/Thailand railroad:

At one camp out in the bush I was on a work party bringing in firewood for the camp cookhouse. The Thai conductor supplying the wood stacked it and our job was to load it into barges for transport to camp. The wood was, of necessity, dry and its bark lifting off. Often scorpions sheltered beneath. They were grey fellows, about six inches long, and packed an extremely painful sting which would prostrate for several hours anyone unfortunate enough to suffer one. We knew of no way of alleviating the pain.

The wood was passed in a chain from the stack to the barge and by about the fourth man any scorpion present would have been disturbed so from there on in the chain one stood at risk. On the occasion I have in mind, I was near to a man who got stung. Very soon an angry weal developed, moving up his arm, and the stricken man had the unhappy prospect of several hours of misery.

An ancient Thai man was squatting on his haunches watching us work. He saw the accident, and coming over he gently lifted the man's arm up and mimed a stroking action downwards. On reaching the victim's fingers, he simulated a throwing-away flick with his own fingers. He did this for about five minutes, by which time the pain in the injured arm was all but dissipated to a mild dullness which itself soon passed. I had learned enough Thai to hold a simple conversation so I spoke to him to thank him, equally to seek an explanation of this miracle. Maybe it was just something he could do, and it seemed to me it was bordering on rudeness that I should be inquisitive about this.

SEA URCHIN INJURIES

The following treatment for sea urchin injury was described by Dr Per Falkenberg of the University of Copenhagen: 'While bathing in the Caribbean sea, a 36-year-old woman trod on a sea urchin and several spines entered her forefoot. Immediately she was treated in the manner employed by the local fishermen: the spines were crushed *in situ* by knocking the sites of entrance with a stone. Thereafter freshly voided urine was poured on the wound. She had no pain in the foot after this treatment and could walk immediately. One month after the accident there were no external signs of injury and X-ray films did not show any foreign bodies.'

JELLYFISH STINGS

Miss Monica Finan from Formby writes: 'On Greek islands tourists used to be advised to use urine for the pain of jellyfish stings. A baby's urine (or a soiled nappy) was considered best.' The active ingredient would be the ammonia-containing waste product urea, and indeed there are now commercial preparations for bites and stings currently available also containing ammonia.

Stitch

The cause of the crippling pain in the upper abdomen, usually on the right side following exercise, commonly known as a stitch, is a medical mystery. It can be precipitated by eating a large meal but more frequently by exercise that jolts the body like running on hard ground or in boggy countryside. It is particularly common in horse (and even more so camel) riders but rare in swimmers, skaters and cyclists.

The most plausible theory is that a stitch is caused by stretching of the ligaments which hold the gut in place, and on these grounds the following remedies are proposed, first prevention and then treatment:

Prevention: No food or water should be taken for two to four hours before exercise. In addition, the abdominal muscles should be strengthened by lying down with raised knees and hips and raising the head towards the upper chest.

Treatment: Stand on your head.

Styes

A stye is caused by blockage of the hair follicle of an eyelash behind which a small collection of infected material accumulates. The usual medical treatment is with an antibiotic cream, but there are a variety of home remedies that are equally or more effective.

Hot compresses: Hot compresses are a reliable way of bringing the stye to a head. The simplest method is to apply to the eyelash cotton wool or a piece of gauze that has been dipped in hot water to which salt has been added.

Saliva: The anti-infective properties of saliva make it a suitable treatment for styes. Regular applications of early morning spittle to a stye in its early stages will prevent it developing.

Water: Mrs Hazel Hall from Lancashire reports: 'As a child of eleven or twelve I suffered greatly with styes and my eyes were rarely free from them. As soon as one had cleared up another appeared. My aunt recommended I should bathe my eyes in urine. Both my mother and I were immensely relieved when a friend of the family, a Swiss doctor, advised me instead to plunge my face in a washbasin of cold water each morning and open my eyes under water three times. I did so and have not suffered since.'

Wedding ring: This remedy is particularly interesting because it illustrates so well the difference between the superstitious nonsense of the old wives' tale and the genuine article.

In *Country Things*, published in 1946, Alison Uttley writes that to cure a stye, 'the eyelid is rubbed very gently with pure gold. A wedding ring is used for this without, of course, removing it from the finger which would be unlucky. It has to be drawn three times across the afflicted eye. My mother often touched somebody's stye with her ring and even the most obstinate one disappeared within a few hours.'

Mrs Mary Goodby from Chester puts the record straight about 'this excellent treatment'. 'In most homes mother's worn, plain gold wedding band is likely to be the only item in the house which is absolutely smooth, without any possible points or corners, non-toxic, very clean due to mum's hands being constantly in water, and a convenient size for the job.'

The precise technique is as follows: 'Hold the ring very firmly by its edge, between finger and thumb. Gently press the opposite half circle onto the affected eyelid while avoiding any possible pressure on the eyeball by performing a sort of gentle scooping action aiming under the stye itself. This causes the stye to empty of pus without hurting the inflamed part around the stye or the eye. An experienced mother could gently turn back the upper or lower eyelid and apply the ring just inside the edge of the lid.'

Taste

The sensation of taste is perceived primarily not through the taste buds in the mouth but rather through the sense of smell in the nose. This major contribution of the sense of smell becomes obvious during a heavy cold when food and drink lose their taste. The contribution of the taste buds in the mouth to 'taste' is limited to four main types—salty, sour, sweet and bitter—evenly distributed around the tongue and palate. Their primary purpose has little to do with the appreciation of food, but rather seems to serve a more basic physiological function. Thus the 'salt' taste is highly sensitive to the amount of salt in the body and induces a craving for the mineral if the blood becomes salt depleted.

There are several types of problem associated with taste, each with their own appropriate home remedy.

Loss of taste: Perceptions of the subtleties of taste decline with age. There is unfortunately little that can be done other than to increase the intensity of the desired sensation—

puddings should be made sweeter, potatoes saltier. It seems sensible also to emphasize the non-taste aspects of food that make it pleasurable. Hot food should be hot, not lukewarm, cold drinks should be cold. Efforts should be made to make food look attractive, and its textures—the slithering avocado, the rawness of *al dente* vegetables—become increasingly important. Some seasoning stimulates the nasal aspects of taste such as horseradish, ginger, cloves, cinammon, pepper and pimento; these should be used more frequently in cooking.

Altered taste: For reasons unknown, one or other of the types of taste buds can come to dominate the others, leading to a persistent and unpleasant salty or sweet taste in the mouth. There is no name for this condition, which must be due to an abnormality of the sensory nerves from the relevant taste buds. There is no ready treatment, but Mr William Boll of Poole suggests: 'The answer is about three teaspoonfuls of salt, partially dissolved in a cup of quite hot water and swilled around the mouth so as to reach every nook and cranny. Hold it in the mouth until the salt solution cools down, then spit out. Repeat until cup is empty. This has to be done two or three times a day and at bedtime. It tastes pretty unpleasant and makes your mouth feel dry and salty, but it is not as bad as the original

251

complaint. This remedy must work by "overwhelming" the abnormal sensation from the salty taste buds.'

Metallic taste: An unpleasant metallic taste in the mouth may be due to prescription eye drops or be the side effect of some other drug.

Bad taste: The obvious cause of a bad taste in the mouth is some form of infection, as described in the section on halitosis (see page 133). When it is associated with a sore mouth and burning, itching lips, it may also be part of a condition known as burning mouth syndrome. There seem to be several possible causes:

Toothpaste
A retired dentist from Cambridge reports that 'in my own case symptoms were caused by toothpaste, and the remedy was a soft brush, child's toothpaste and less zealous, although sufficient, cleaning'. Another reader observes: 'I had used Gibbs SR toothpaste for many years, but burning symptoms developed when I bought a new tube. I presumed that a new ingredient had been added and bought another brand. Comfort was restored and I have had no further problem.'

Dishwasher powder
One woman's symptoms improved after she

stopped using cups and mugs which had been in the dishwasher. 'This seemed to be the answer and I only experience the problem now when I drink out. I then try to rinse my mouth with water as soon as possible.'

Acid regurgitation

Acid regurgitation at night can cause inflammation of the mouth and is promptly controlled by taking acid-suppressant drugs such as Losec.

Food sensitivity

Several foods have been associated with the condition including seedless grapes, bell peppers and raw fruit.

Diabetes

Mrs Brenda Bridge from Wirral: 'I started to suffer from the same symptoms of sore mouth, burning lips, etc. It was only when a great thirst also developed that I was tested and found to have developed diabetes.'

Drugs

The drug captopril, used in the treatment of raised blood pressure, has been implicated.

Teeth

A LOST TOOTH

The Tooth Fairy, it has been calculated, shells out £11 million a year in Britain for 'milk' teeth left under the pillow. Regrettably, her largesse does not extend to adults for whom losing a tooth is a more serious matter, as nature is too parsimonious to provide a replacement. It is therefore all the more important to know that when adult teeth are knocked out there is a high chance of them taking root again if they are quickly replaced in the socket. Pick the tooth up, wash it and just stick it back—making sure that it is the right way round. There is then, according to the *British Medical Journal*, 'a very good chance that it will be retained'.

Regrettably, however, 'many people seem to be alarmed at the prospect of pushing a tooth back into a socket. Someone unable to undertake the task should, however, be capable of storing the tooth in an appropriate solution and looking for a dentist as quickly as possible.' The main reason why a dislodged tooth may fail to reattach is that the cells around its roots dry out and die, so it is important to try to keep it moist—placing it in a cup of milk is apparently ideal—and then get to a dentist within twenty-four hours. The watchword is 'action'.

TOOTHACHE

The cure for toothache is to take some painkillers, gargle with salty warm water and make an appointment to see the dentist as soon as possible. The following remedy from Mr W.K. Ayres of Canterbury recalls the time when people were unable to afford to see the dentist and had no alternative other than to treat themselves.

We lived in a small village seven miles from Dover. My father was a farmer renting his land. In those days, there were no subsidies and he had two successive bad years. The first was a drought—some idiot of a boy set fire to a barn full of corn. By the time the horse-drawn fire brigade from a village two and a half miles away arrived there was nothing left. In direct contrast in the summer of the next year, we had a cloudburst over the village. So you can see we were not very well off and if we had toothache there was no chance of a visit to the dentist.

My mother filled a large saucer with vinegar, sprinkled a good amount of pepper on it and soaked a square of brown paper on it. When it was thoroughly wet, she slapped the square on the cheek nearest the offending tooth and tied it with a large handkerchief. I think it helped because we always slept quite well, but it didn't pay to wriggle one's face in the pillow after the vinegar had evaporated because the brown paper felt like sandpaper.

Brown paper and vinegar feature as a remedy for another ailment—Jack's headache after 'breaking his crown' in the children's nursery rhyme 'Jack and Jill'.

Thrush

Thrush is caused by a yeast—*Candida albicans* —which commonly resides harmlessly in the vagina where it causes no symptoms. Factors that upset the delicate ecology of the vagina will result in the proliferation of the yeast, giving rise to the typical symptoms of itchiness and a white discharge. These include antibiotics taken for infections elsewhere in the body, hormones such as the contraceptive pill and HRT, irritation of the vagina by tampons or insufficient lubrication at intercourse.

The antifungal preparation Canesten is an excellent cure for thrush and can be purchased readily over the counter from the chemist. This is much the best solution for the one-off attack. Those prone to recurrent episodes of thrush should consider the following remedies.

Salt and water: Much relief can be gained by adding a good handful of salt to a bidet or shallow bath and swishing around in the resulting brine.

Vinegar: Vinegar has a similar acidity to the vaginal secretions which, it is believed, control the proliferation of the yeast. Vaginal acidity can be restored by douching in a mixture of four teaspoonfuls of vinegar to half a litre of warm water.

Hairdryer: Drying the vaginal area with a hairdryer rather than a towel will minimize irritation of the region.

Clothes: Warm and damp environments promote the growth of yeasts, so it is advised that loose-fitting cotton underwear should be worn close to the skin. Cutting the gusset out of tights promotes circulation of air to the genital area.

Live yoghurt: Live yoghurt contains the harmless bug *Lactobacillus* and helps to suppress the proliferation of *Candida* in the vagina. It is advised that a pot of live yoghurt eaten every day will control the irritation, and a small amount on the tip of a tampon can be introduced directly into the vagina.

Tinnitus

'My ears whistle and buzz continuously day and night. I can say I am leading a wretched life,' poor old Beethoven complained about his tinnitus. Had it been available at the time, a Walkman mini-stereo might have helped for, as Aristotle observed, 'Buzzing in the ears ceases when a greater sound drives out the lesser.' Tinnitus is the amplification of the noise that can be induced by placing both hands over the ears. Many people experience it, especially those like Beethoven who have some form of hearing impairment. Tinnitus can come to dominate their lives. There is no medical treatment, though many who suffer from tinnitus are helped by consulting a hearing therapist who can advise on means of minimizing the symptoms. The possibilities for home remedies are as follows:

'A greater sound drives out the lesser': Mr H. Beech from Cheshunt describes his technique for getting rid of the tinnitus that prevents his sleeping. 'The tinnitus can be masked by a small portable radio. When it is set to the FM band, the frequency between 104 to 108 MHz produces a sound like a rushing of air in the trees. This is supplemented by an under-pillow speaker plugged into the earpiece socket.' Alternatively, Mrs D. Webber from Weston reports that if she turns the radio up very loud for forty-five minutes—her preference is for Radio 5—and then turns it off, she finds that she 'can hear a pin drop' and is able to drift off to sleep.

'Beating the drum': Mr F. Byrne from Salford finds he can hasten the departure of his tinnitus with a yoga exercise known as 'beating the drum': 'Using the forefingers, close the flaps of each ear and then beat on the nails of the forefingers with the next digit.'

Massage: Massaging near the ears can also help, as one reader reports: 'I can find an area in front of each ear which if pressed exacerbates the tinnitus. If I then massage these areas I often get relief—not immediately but some time afterwards.' Other recommended massage sites include behind the ear lobe in front of the mastoid bone and 'the depression formed in front of the ears when the mouth is open'.

The Tongue

The tongue's appearance is widely believed to be a reliable indicator of general health. If the tongue is clear and shiny, all is well, but if it is furred then all is not well. Traditional Chinese medicine goes even further, interpreting flabbiness as suggestive of a gastric ulcer, paleness of hay fever and a yellow coating as a sign of bowel problems.

These distinctions are a bit too subtle to be reliable, which is not to say that the tongue may not at times have a very bizarre appearance and produce quite distressing symptoms.

Black hairy tongue: A 'black hairy tongue' is a considerable nuisance as the sufferer has the persistent sensation that the back of the palate is being tickled. The 'hairiness' is due to elongation of the cells at the back of the tongue, while the black colour is caused by pigment-forming bacteria. Dr Joanna Zakrzewski, senior lecturer at St Bartholomew's Hospital in London, recommends 'tongue brushing and scraping and an increase in roughage in the diet'. Further, and as with the treatment of mouth ulcers, several readers recommend the cleansing properties of pineapple regularly consumed.

Geographical tongue: This is so called because the tongue looks like an ever-changing map of the world. Red patches surrounded by a white border resembling the shape of continents develop on the surface of the tongue, then fade away to reappear in a different form. Its cause is not known and doctors tend not to be interested, but sufferers maintain that the condition is anything but trivial as it considerably interferes with the pleasures of eating, particularly astringent foods like fruit and tomatoes.

Mrs C.A. Williams from Nottinghamshire describes a treatment that worked for her: 'My tongue was coated with huge sore circles, and just as one disappeared another one arrived. People were amazed when I showed them. My sister was horrified at the state of my tongue and rushed me to her local pharmacist. He was most helpful and said that I was deficient in all the B vitamins. I came away with a large supply, one to be taken each day. I am pleased to say there has been a huge improvement. The sore circles do recur, but with the tablets and the mouthwash Corsodyl, they go quite quickly.'

Mr Stanley Rubin from Manchester suggests the following mouthwash which he describes as having 'come about from trial and error by consultation between myself and a friendly pharmacist'. It is, he says, 'helpful and soothing whenever an attack of the discomfort arises. Take 10 ml of 20 per cent solution of chlorhexidine with 10 ml concentrated peppermint emulsion and 10 ml chloroform water. Add purified water to 1000 ml.'

Warts

Warts can occur virtually anywhere on the body, but they are most common on the hands and fingers, where they are unsightly, and on the feet where they are known as verrucas and can be painful. They are caused by a virus— the human papillomavirus, or HPV—and can spread from one site of the body to another. They are probably only slightly infective and so difficult to 'catch' from someone else, though it is commonly believed that verrucas may be acquired from communal swimming baths.

The only interesting thing about warts is how to get rid of them, and here there are essentially two options. The first is to obtain from the chemist (or doctor on prescription) a paint or gel which contains salicyclic acid which when regularly applied over a period of three months usually manages to eradicate them. The recommended technique is first to soak the wart in warm water for a couple of minutes, dry it and then carefully apply the paint and allow it to dry. This produces an elastic film over the wart which should be carefully removed and the procedure repeated the following day. The surface of the wart should then be rubbed with a pumice stone or piece of sandpaper once a week.

The second standard therapy is to burn the warts off with liquid nitrogen; this acts much more quickly. The treatment is usually only performed by skin specialists in the local hospital, and there is usually a waiting list of three months or so before being seen. So either way, it takes quite a time to get rid of a wart—time enough to try one of several simple remedies.

More than any other remedies described in this book, those for warts are probably the least convincing and most vulnerable to the charge 'quackery'. Their efficacy is very difficult to assess because most—perhaps 75 per cent—of warts are likely to disappear of their own accord without any treatment within a couple of years. Thus virtually any remedy will seem to work for some people because the wart's disappearance will coincide with the time it was going to resolve anyhow.

Many traditional remedies are indeed 'quackery', such as the advice that the wart should be rubbed with a piece of meat which should then be buried 'secretly', or the advice to wash the wart in the light of the moon. None the less, despite their superstitious nature, such remedies could still work because warts are one of those human conditions that are wholly amenable to suggestion—that is, if the person believes strongly enough in the remedy, the warts will indeed disappear.

Thus, Dr Christopher McEwen, a skin specialist from Louisiana, reports: 'I have treated a couple of children who could not tolerate freezing [with liquid nitrogen]. So I gave them a harmless substance to use and impressed upon them that it was a very strong medicine that would knock out the warts. And it worked.'

In a similar vein, Dr Nicholas Spanos, a

263

psychologist from Ottawa, describes the effect of encouraging those with warts to spirit their warts away with visual imagery. 'We tell patients to imagine their warts are shrinking, that they can feel the tingling as their warts dissolve and their skin becomes clear. Those who report really vivid imagery are more likely to lose their warts than those who say their imagery was weak.'

The most frequently recommended of the many suggested home remedies for warts include the following:

Saliva: Saliva has anti-infective properties which may be effective against the papillomavirus. 'My method is to apply saliva to the offending spot. I first discovered the remedy by nibbling away at a wart on the knuckle of one of my fingers. Warts outside the nibbling range have to be dealt with by wetting the tip of the finger and applying the saliva in that manner.' Mr K.S.M. Sears from Surbiton.

Several contributors report that the best effects are obtained with saliva obtained first thing in the morning—'fasting spittle'.

Broad bean pods: 'Some years ago I had a verruca which persisted for over two years despite the best efforts of my doctor and the fact that I had developed a slight limp. When listening to the radio one day I heard a man saying he had been similarly afflicted and his doctor had advised him to use broad bean pods rubbed on night and morning. I immediately started doing this—it being the right season for broad beans—and within three weeks the verruca disappeared, never to return.' Mrs V. Haslam from Kent.

Banana: A variant of the broad bean cure is to use the inside of a banana skin, as described by Mrs Olwyn Wych from Cheshire: 'Forty years ago I read how warts could be "removed" by rubbing with the inside of a banana skin. As I had a large wart (half an inch across) on my wrist at the base of my thumb, I was prepared to give this a try. A couple of weeks later I noticed that it had gone. I have passed this remedy on to several colleagues over the years and it has proved to be successful.'

Dr Livia Warszawer Schvarcz describes the practicalities in the *Journal of Plastic and Reconstructive Surgery*. 'The inside of a banana skin is attached to the wart once daily after washing. After one week of treatment the wart becomes softer and the pain diminishes. After two weeks, shrinkage of the wart becomes obvious. After maximal treatment of six weeks, the wart completely disappears.'

Dettol: 'A cure for verrucas that has never once failed in the thirty-six years I have been recommending it, is to soak the foot each night in water as hot as you can bear it then dab with undiluted Dettol. The verruca dropped out in a week.' Mr W. Cassel from Sittingbourne.

Suggestion: Sometimes suggestion works and sometimes it does not. Mr R.E. Paul from Oxfordshire recalls:

As a small boy in the twenties my hands were covered with warts which my mother was convinced were caused by my handling of milk churns on a farm where we frequently helped with the milking. Conventional treatment, mainly burning with a caustic pencil, had only limited success so another country remedy was tried. My mother gave me a small piece of steak and instructed me to rub this on the warts and bury the steak in the garden at night, revealing to no one the site of the interment.

This treatment also failed, and on the advice of a neighbour, mother then took me to see a local countryman who was known as a wart charmer. The old gentleman consulted his calendar and asked me to come back on a certain date, the night of the full moon. On the appointed night I presented myself apprehensively and was taken out into the garden where Mr Hunt took my hands in his and fingered all the warts while gazing up at the moon and muttering some inaudible invocation. He then said to me, 'Don't thank me and don't pay me or else the charm will not work.' I did not believe this rigmarole for a minute, but within a few days all the warts had completely disappeared, never to return.

Wind

The facility to expel unwanted gas from the gut, either upwards or downwards, is essential for human happiness. The great virtue of belching is that it permits pockets of air trapped in the stomach to eructate upwards, rather than having to travel the length of the intestine before being released. Though the expulsion of those intestinal gases is essential to health, it is always possible to have too much of a good thing and the overproduction of wind can pose serious social problems.

The case of a 28-year-old man, currently the acknowledged world record-holder for the passage of flatus—140 times in one day—is instructive. He found it difficult to persuade the medical fraternity to take his problem seriously until his plight came to the attention of Dr Michael Levitt of the University of Minnesota. The main source of intestinal gases are the fermentation by bacteria in the colon of undigested food residues; hence excessive wind is likely to be due to failure to absorb certain types of food. Dr Levitt found that his patient was intolerant of the sugar lactose present in milk and dairy products. The elimination of lactose-containing foods had a dramatic effect in reducing the frequency of passing flatus to twenty-five times a day, though this is slightly higher than the 'normal' average figure of fourteen times a day.

A different approach is necessary for those whose wind gets trapped in the colon causing abdominal discomfort and distension. Charcoal tablets, available from the chemist, absorb excess gas and can provide short-term relief. The best method of dispersing trapped wind, however, was discovered by accident by a patient admitted to hospital with toxic megacolon—an inflammatory condition of the bowel, which becomes grossly distended with vast quantities of gas.

While trying to make himself more comfortable, the patient adopted the Mecca position—kneeling on the bed bent forward with his arms stretched out in front and his bottom sticking up in the air. In this position he passed a monumental quantity of flatus 'which continued for several minutes'. He immediately felt more comfortable, so he repeated this manoeuvre several times 'with similar results'. He described his experience to his astonished surgeon, Mr M.Z. Panos of the University of Birmingham, who measured his abdominal girth and discovered that he had indeed become a lot slimmer. 'Over the next fortnight his condition gradually improved at which point he was discharged fully recovered,' comments Dr Panos.

It has subsequently become standard practice for surgeons to prescribe the 'Mecca position' in such circumstances, thus avoiding much unnecessary surgery. The same technique is also likely to be of value for those with trapped or excess wind for other reasons such as constipation or an overconsumption of beans.

Finally, it is helpful to know that when visiting friends and relations, lighting a match after a visit to the toilet will eliminate any sulphurous smells left behind. Solicitous hosts will leave a box of matches in the 'little room' for this purpose, though Swan are apparently more effective than safety matches.

Acknowledgements

This book could not have been written without the help of many readers of the *Daily Telegraph*. They include:

Mr J. Aaron, G.D. Adams, Mrs Ann Ainsworth, Mr H.J. Allen, Mr W.S. Annable, Mrs P. .M. Ansell, Mrs Elizabeth Ardill, P Austin, Mrs Peggy Auton, W.K. Ayers, Mr Ron Ayerst, Mr John Bainbridge, Mr A.L. Baker, Mr F. Baley, Mrs Marion Banyard, Miss M.D. Barnes, Mrs J. Barton, Mr John Bassett, J.C. Beard, Mr Geoffrey Bellis, Margaret Bellord, Mr Edward Bennett, Mrs Constance Benton, Mrs Pamela Betts, Ann Birks, Mrs Daphne Blacock, W.D. Blake, Mrs Bet Bolt, Mrs Vivien Bolton, Hilary Bonye, Mrs P.R. Booth, Mr Derek Boxall, Mirja Boyd, Angela Breckon, A.C.J. Brent-Good, Mr Norman Bromley, Irene Broughton, Mr Ernest Brown, Mr John Brown, Mrs Nancy Brown, Mrs Julie Buchanan, Mrs Penny Bullivant, Mrs J.L. Butler, N.W. Byrne, Mrs M.D. Cameron, Margaret Cameron, Mr John Campbell, Mrs Evelyn Careless, Miss M.E. Caryfield, Mrs P.M. Caseley, Mrs C. Castellan, Mr Robert Cawley, B.M. Charratt, Mrs Constance Clark, Mavis Clark, Miss R.T. Clark, Carolyn Clarke, Dr J.C. Clarke, Vera Clarke, Mr Claxton,

Commander R.H. Colby RN, Mr Roy Collins, Helen Cooper, Colonel V.J.C. Cooper, Mrs S. Cortis, Mrs Mirren Coxon, G.W.J. Crawford, Mrs Sally Crinean, Mrs Christine Crosland, Mrs Barbara Daniels, Mrs I.E. Darnel, Professor D.A.M. Davies, J.H. Davies, Roberta Davies, Louise Dawson, Mrs Shirley De Ath, Mrs Julie De Vile, Mrs Margaret Dent, J. Derlien, Mrs Drummond Crabbe, W.I. Drysdale, Mrs Irene Duncan, Margaret Edy, Mary Elliott, Mrs D.M. Evans, Irene Evans, Mr Brian Evers, Mr John Eyton-Jones, Mr Alan Fenemore, Mr David Fairburn, Mr P.J. Fenerty, Mrs E. Field, J.H. Fisher, Mrs Mary Flint, Miss Marie Flower, Mrs Pat Franklin, Mr Derek Fraylen, D. Fryer, Miss B.J. Gadd, Mr Norman Gardiner, Mrs M.S. Geering, Mrs F.A.B. George, Mr John Gilbert, Mrs T.M. Godber, Mrs D.P. Gomez, R.A. Goodbar, Mrs Mary Goodby, Mrs S.R. Goodman, Mrs Iris Goodreid, Mr Paul Goriup, Mr Basil Gotto, Mrs Audrey Graham, Mr Alan Grant, Mr John Granville, M. Gray, Mr Cyril Green, Mr John Green, G. Green, Mr S.J. Green, Mr S. Greening-Jackson, Joan Greenup, Margaret Griffin, Mrs K.D. Hall, Mrs Margareta Hallam, A.G. Halligey, Professor J.M.T. Hamilton-Miller, Mr James Hannay, Miss M.L.B. Harberd, Florence Harrison, Dorothy Hedley, Mrs Pauline Hemsley, C. Hepworth, Mrs P. Hester, Mrs V.J.B. Hibbert, Mrs M. Hill, Mrs David Hilton, Mr Robert Hilton,

Mrs Geraldine Hobson, J. Hockley, Mrs J. Holland, Mrs E.C. Hood, Mr U.G. Huggins, A.W. Hutchinson, H.H.F Hutchinson, Mrs Ann Irwin, Miss Barbara Ivey, Mr Morrison James, Mr T.P.M. Jenkins, Sheila Jennings, Mr R.D. Jephcott, Mr Stephen Jessop, Mrs Elise Johnston, Mrs Ruby Johnston, Mr J. Jolley, G.A. Jolly, Mrs Elizabeth Jones, Mrs Jill Jones, Mrs M.L. Jones, Mrs Diana Joslin, Irene Katchourin, Mr Michael Keef, Mr Niall Kennedy, Thea Kennedy, Mr W.T. Kermode, Mrs Ruth Kershaw, Mrs Sheila Kewlil, Mary King, Mrs N.M. King, Mrs E.M. Kirby, Margaret Kirtz, Mr Hugh Langford, Mrs Jill Leaberry, Helen Lee, Gabriel Lewis, Mr Rory Linden-Kelly, Mr Alan Lord, Mr Roy Lowe, Angela Lyle, Miss Eileen Lynch, Kathleen Macdonald, Patricia MacLaren Butler, Angela Maclean, Mrs Margaret Malloy, Mrs Edna Markiewicz, Mrs E.M. Martin, Mr John Maslen, P. Mason, Lt-Col. H.P.S. Massy, Mr Matthews, Jill McAnee, Mrs Stella McCandless, Belinda Mead, Mr Douglas Meaden, Mrs Jill Mendel, Mrs Daphne Meryon, Mrs Barbara Middleton, Mr Peter Miles, Dr R.M. Miller, Mr Clive Mills, Brenda Mold, Mr Alastair Monroe, Mrs Jane Morgan, Mr J. Morley, Mrs H.M. Morrish, F.A. Murphy, Rowena Nesbitt, Mr Jeremy Nichols, Mrs Mary Nichols, M. Nichols. J.A. Nicol, Mrs I. Northfield, Miss Patricia O'Driscoll, Sheila O'Reilly, Mr E. Oliver, Mrs Pamela Orpen, Mr

H. Orr, Ms J. Orritt, Mr Jack Palmer, Mr T.W Palmer, Mr Peter Parr, Mary Parsons, Mr John S. Paterson, Dr M.F Paterson, R.E. Paul, Miss Jean A. Peale, T..R. Pearce, Mr Clifton Pender, Mr G.L. Phillipson, Mrs Dinah Pichersfill, Mrs Joanne Pierce, Mrs G.S. Pink, Mrs Belinda Platt, Miss A. Powell, Mr G.V. Pride, Dr T.R.F. Raw, Mrs E. Redgrave, Mr Tom Rees-Jones, Evelyn Rice, Mr D.J. Richards, W. Robins, Miss Edith Rolfe, Jean Rooney, Mrs Mary Rosewarne, Mr H. Row, Peggy Rowell, Mr F.W. Sanders, Mr B.R. Sandwell, Mr K.S.M. Sears, F. Seiflow, Mr John Shelton, Mrs P Sherwood, P.G. Shingler, Mrs Ellene Simmonds, D.J. Simpson, S.A. Skinner, Mrs Jean Slater, Mrs Angela Smith, Dr John Smith, Mr K.E. Smith, Mr K.R. Smith, M.D. Smith, Mrs R.J. Stanbury, Mrs Mary Stay, Mr J. Stewart, Mr Paul Stickley, Mr Andrew Stronach, Mr David Strudwick, Mrs A.J. Swaine, Thelma Swales, Mrs J.N. Swinscow, Mrs E.M. Tanfield, C. Tarleton, Mrs E. Taylor, Mrs Frances Taylor, R.C.N. Thomas, Mrs Marianne Ticehurst, S.J. Tims, Mr Paul Tunbridge, Mrs Sylva Usher, Janet Valentine, J.I. Visser, Isobel Wagg, Dr E.S. Waight, A. Warburton, Mr E.O. Wardroper, G.T. Warner, Margaret Watson, Mrs D. Watt, Mr Chris Webb, Mrs Marjorie Wells, Mrs P. Whetton, Mrs A. White, Mrs M.E. Whitehead, Kathleen Whiteman, Mrs Margaret Wilkins, Mrs E. Wilkinson, Mr Martin Willcocks, Mrs

Barbara Willett, Mrs Kathleen Williams, Linda Williams, Mr Allan Wilson, Eileen Wilson, Yvonne Wilson, Mrs Vivien Womersley, Mrs Marguerite Wood, Shelagh Wood, Mrs Evelyn Woodfield, Miss I.E. Woolford, Mrs Rosemary Wray, Lady Patsy Yardley, Mrs Gogi Younger, Mrs Joan Zetterholm.

We hope you have enjoyed this Large Print book. Other Chivers Press or Thorndike Press Large Print books are available at your library or directly from the publishers.

For more information about current and forthcoming titles, please call or write, without obligation, to:

Chivers Press Limited
Windsor Bridge Road
Bath BA2 3AX
England
Tel. (01225) 335336

OR

Thorndike Press
295 Kennedy Memorial Drive
Waterville
Maine 04901
USA

All our Large Print titles are designed for easy reading, and all our books are made to last.